# MMR AND AUTISM

Speculation that MMR – the combined vaccine against measles, mumps and rubella – may be a cause of autism in children has provoked fierce controversy and widespread anxiety.

Though medical opinion is overwhelmingly in favour of MMR, the campaign against the vaccine has made many parents worried and confused. Both professionals and parents struggle to cope with the resulting anxieties and fears and find it difficult to get a balanced account of the issues.

In *MMR and Autism* Michael Fitzpatrick, a general practitioner who is also the parent of an autistic child, explains why he believes the anti-MMR campaign is misguided in a way that will reassure parents considering vaccination and also relieve the continued anxieties of parents of autistic children. At the same time the book provides healthcare professionals and health studies students with an accessible overview of a contemporary health and media issue with significant policy implications.

**Michael Fitzpatrick** is a general practitioner working in Hackney, London.

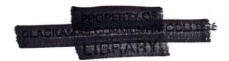

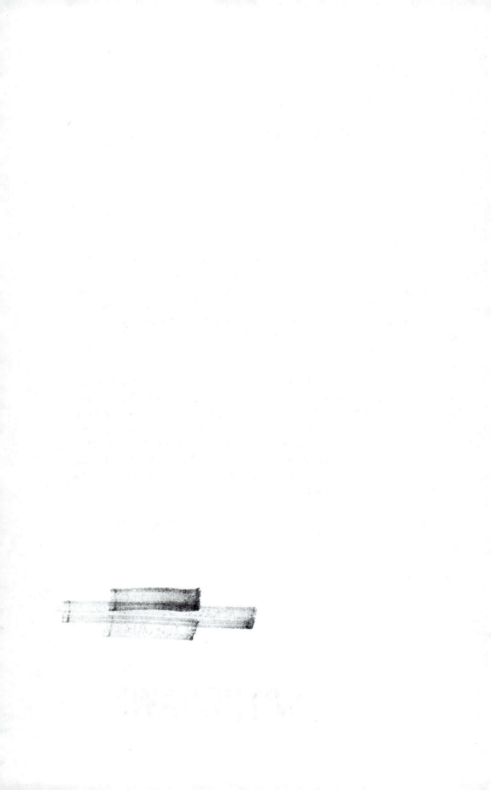

# MMR AND AUTISM

## What parents need to know

## *Michael Fitzpatrick*

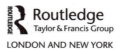

**Routledge**
Taylor & Francis Group

LONDON AND NEW YORK

First published in 2004 by Routledge
11 New Fetter Lane, London EC4P 4EE

Simultaneously published in the USA and Canada
by Routledge
29 West 35th Street, New York, NY 10001

*Routledge is an imprint of the Taylor & Francis Group*

© 2004 Michael Fitzpatrick

Typeset in Times by J&L Composition, Filey, North Yorkshire
Printed and bound in Great Britain by Biddles Ltd,
Guildford and King's Lynn

*British Library Cataloguing in Publication Data*
A catalogue record for this book is available from the British Library

*Library of Congress Cataloging in Publication Data*
A catalogue record has been requested

ISBN 0–415–32178–6
ISBN 0–415–32179–4

# CONTENTS

# PREFACE

I happened to be doing the baby clinic on the day in February 1998 when the story broke about a link between the MMR vaccine and autism. In the lull before the clinic got underway I rang the 'immunisation hotline' – a service that was advertised in a yellowing poster on the noticeboard – to find out the official response to what seemed likely to become a major scare. Visualising a red phone ringing and flashing on some distant government desk, I was surprised to find the call answered promptly by our friendly local community paediatrician.

She tried to reassure me that a detailed refutation of the paper published in *The Lancet* by gastroenterologist Andrew Wakefield and others, which suggested a link between the MMR vaccine and autism mediated by inflammatory bowel disease, would be circulated shortly and that this should soothe parental anxieties. I indicated my fears that, even if Dr Wakefield were wrong, a scare of this sort might still result in a serious setback for the national immunisation campaign. Nearly six years later, it looks as if my forebodings were justified. It is indeed now almost universally accepted that Dr Wakefield has not made a convincing case for a link between MMR and autism, but the rate of uptake of the vaccine nationally has fallen below 85 per cent – 10 per cent lower than the target required to prevent outbreaks of measles. In our clinic, in common with many inner London areas, uptake is now below 75 per cent.

My first response to the MMR–autism link was as a family doctor fielding enquiries from worried parents. At the time I was beginning work on a book, subsequently published as *The Tyranny of Health* (Fitzpatrick 2001), which included a discussion of the impact of scares around issues such as HIV/AIDS, sun-related skin cancer, 'mad cow disease' and thrombosis linked to the oral contraceptive pill. I included a brief account of the MMR–autism scare, noting how it 'led to a period of intensive and prolonged discussions in the baby clinic as parents agonised over the decision whether to have their baby vaccinated, baffled and confused by contradictory medical opinions' (Fitzpatrick 2001: 19).

But I had another interest in the MMR–autism hypothesis: my son James had been diagnosed as autistic in 1994 at the age of two. The controversy over MMR sent us back to examine his immunisation records and brought back painful memories of the prolonged process of discovery that led to his diagnosis.

At Christmas 1993, James, then just 18 months old, had delighted his grandma by responding to her commands to point to his head, nose and tummy. He began to say a few words and family snaps confirm an ever-smiling, delightful, playful toddler. But over the next few months the words stopped and he seemed to drift slowly away. He appeared subdued and withdrawn, he avoided eye contact and seemed not to hear when people spoke to him. When we tried to play with him, he would seem uninterested and wander off, apparently happy to be on his own, walking around on tiptoes, jumping up and down, flapping his hands and making squeaking noises.

For weeks, my wife Mary and I came up with numerous explanations for James' behaviour: he had a viral illness and was teething (he did and he was); he was upset because Mary was away for a few days. We found ourselves making more and more of an effort to engage him. We also noticed that his brother Michael, 16 months older, appeared to have given up trying to get James to play with him.

My period of denial ended one day in the library at Homerton Hospital, where I had gone to look up some problem that had come up at the surgery. Or was I there for that reason? I soon found myself poring over a dusty textbook of child psychiatry in a section headed 'infantile autism'. At almost the same moment, Mary – a university lecturer – had found the same condition in her library. We immediately embarked on a frantic quest for expert confirmation of the diagnosis. But, by then, we knew.

A glance at James' Child Health Record confirmed that he had received a full set of immunisations in his first year and MMR at 14 months (he had his 'pre-school booster' jabs slightly late, at the age of 5). We did not notice any adverse effects from any of these immunisations. In retrospect, it emerges that we first became concerned about James' behaviour about four months after his MMR, although at the time we did not make any particular connection between these events. His brother also had a full course of vaccinations – without incident – and he has not turned out to be autistic.

When we discovered that James was autistic we spent many months in a state of shock, grief, anxiety and anger: indeed, elements of all these emotions persist to this day. We can well understand how parents whose babies first manifested features of autism shortly after receiving MMR could attribute a causal role to the vaccine. When you are in a state of distress at discovering your baby is autistic, you cling to any explanation on offer. However, although it may provide some comfort to have something or somebody to blame, such emotional responses are unlikely to find the right target.

On thinking further about the MMR–autism thesis after the news broke, I was sceptical about it for a number of reasons. Autism has been recognised since the 1940s (and historical accounts suggest that, even if it was not previously recognised, it certainly existed) (Houston, Frith 2000). As measles and, later, MMR immunisations only came into use from the 1960s onwards, this is an unlikely general explanation for autism. Furthermore, although the hypothesis suggests that the attenuated form of the measles virus present in MMR may cause autism, measles itself has never been shown to do this (unlike the rubella virus which may cause autism as part of the congenital rubella syndrome). Given that MMR has now been in use in many countries for many years, it seems likely that if it were a significant cause of autism this would have been noted elsewhere. Yet the question of a link with MMR has only arisen in Britain (although the scare has subsequently spread to other English-speaking countries). As autism commonly becomes apparent in the second year of life – at around the same time as the MMR is given – it would not be surprising if an association between the two events arose by chance.

Nevertheless, I was aware that having had James immunised, it was possible that my own reaction, as well as being vulnerable to the desire to blame others, might also have been pointed in a contrary direction by a wish to deny that I had permitted a procedure that may have contributed to his condition. So I made it my business to read Dr Wakefield's *Lancet* paper very carefully. My first response was one of amazement that such an insubstantial and speculative report should have had such an impact. Although the authors admitted that they 'did not prove a causal association' between MMR and autism, it would be more accurate to say that they did not provide *any* evidence of a causal relationship. They simply reported the conviction of the parents of eight of the 12 children in the study that there was a link between MMR and the onset of behavioural problems. (It subsequently emerged [see Chapter 7] that these parents had previously been exposed both to Dr Wakefield's view that the measles vaccine could cause inflammatory bowel disease and to anti-immunisation campaigners' belief that MMR could cause autism.) Putting this together with the implausibility of the postulated mechanism through which MMR was said to produce autism, I was unimpressed with the theory that MMR was a factor in causing autism – in James or any other child.

As the intensity of the MMR–autism controversy fluctuated from the late 1990s onwards, there was a striking divergence between the perception of the issue among scientists and doctors on the one hand, and among parents and the wider public on the other. Given the serious issues at stake, a number of expert committees, including the Medical Research Council in Britain, and the Academy of Pediatrics and the Institute of Medicine in the USA, examined – in impressive detail – the case for the MMR–autism link, and categorically rejected it (see Chapter 9).

The fact that a long list of bodies representing the medical and allied professions made similar judgements might be attributed to the conformist character of such institutions (DH 2002). But scrupulously independent authorities also came to the same conclusion.

Edited by clinical pharmacologist Professor Joe Collier, and published by the Consumers' Association, the *Drug and Therapeutics Bulletin* receives no funding from pharmaceutical companies and carries no advertising. It is regarded by many doctors as one of the most reliable sources of information about drugs and other medical interventions. In its assessment of the MMR vaccine, it concluded that there was 'no convincing evidence that MMR vaccine causes, or facilitates development of, either inflammatory bowel disease or autism' (Anon 2003: 29). (It emphasised that 'the weight of published evidence argues overwhelmingly in favour of MMR vaccine as the most effective and safest way of protecting children from measles, mumps and rubella' and found that 'there was no good reason' to opt for separate vaccines.)

Although those who inhabit the worlds of science and medicine may have been virtually unanimous in rejecting the case against MMR, the persistence of the controversy resulted in a gradual decline in uptake of the vaccine. While some parents rejected MMR, others opted to give each of the components as separate vaccines as a compromise position. Even when parents have opted to give their children MMR, the decision was often fraught with anxiety.

Despite the overwhelming weight of scientific evidence against Dr Wakefield's hypothesis, his preliminary 'early report' – based on a series of a dozen cases – has gravely damaged a nationwide immunisation programme that had become firmly established over the preceding decade. Dr Wakefield's paper appears to be a dramatic example of the butterfly effect celebrated in chaos theory, in which the flutter of tiny wings on one continent is amplified around the planet to produce a tidal wave on some distant shore. Perhaps more prosaically, the Wakefield effect may be understood as an illustration of the impact of a particularly potent health scare in a society pervaded by an enhanced consciousness of risk. In this febrile climate, the MMR scare has provoked a revolt of the anxious middle classes against a government that has tried doggedly but increasingly unsuccessfully to hold the line against a set of values (notably those of consumer sovereignty and choice) that it has done much to promote.

While I feared that the MMR scare might have a lasting effect on vaccine uptake, I did not anticipate that it would have such a big impact on the world of autism. However, more and more parents of autistic children were drawn into the campaign against MMR. Soon more than 1,000 were engaged in litigation against the vaccine manufacturers in a class action that dragged on to the end of 2003 when the Legal Services Commission finally decided to withdraw Legal Aid, and plans for the case to be heard in April 2004 were abandoned. Despite this setback, the legal campaign is likely to continue in some form, although given the lack of evidence for the parents' claims it is destined to end in disappointment and disillusionment. The link-up between parents of autistic children and the anti-immunisation campaigns is a great misfortune of recent years. It will not benefit our children and, if immunisation rates continue to fall, it may well damage other people's children.

The key moment in my decision to become more actively involved in the MMR–autism controversy came in early 2002 when the mother of a boy newly diagnosed with autism came into the surgery to tell me how guilty she felt that, by agreeing for him to have MMR, she had helped to render him autistic. Parents of autistic children have enough difficulties without having to shoulder an additional and utterly unwarranted burden of guilt over MMR.

My aim in writing *MMR and Autism: What parents need to know* is, first, to make whatever contribution I can to relieving parental angst about MMR. Through examining the thesis itself and providing an account of what is known about it from a range of sources, I want to reassure parents faced with decisions about vaccinations that they have nothing to fear in MMR and every reason to welcome the protection it affords their children. I particularly want to reassure parents of children with autism that they have no cause to blame themselves over MMR. There is no good evidence to support a causative link between MMR and autism and strong evidence that it protects children against serious infectious diseases.

It may be that the tide is already turning back in favour of MMR – I certainly hope so. Even if that is the case, we are left with what is possibly an even bigger issue. How on earth did this happen? Something needs explaining here, and not just for the benefit of parents. We have to explain how it has come about that a significant section of middle-class opinion in particular has come to reject, or at least seriously question, immunisation, regarded by many as one of the great achievements of medical science; that scientists and doctors, as well as politicians, have proved so ineffectual in defending the immunisation programme; that many parents are asserting their right to expose their children (and other people's children) to significant risks of serious diseases. Only by exploring the wider culture of our time can we begin to explain how such an irrational campaign as that launched against MMR could acquire a substantial influence in society. That is what I also seek to do in this book.

Given the often-contested status of scientific authority in the MMR controversy, I should declare my own qualifications. I have a Bachelor's degree in physiology and basic medical qualifications. I have no post-graduate qualifications in any discipline specifically relevant to MMR or autism. I have practised for 20 years as a GP in East London. As a GP I receive incentive payments for achieving immunisation targets. In our practice of six partners, I calculate that in 2002 we received about 95p each for every immunisation carried out. Unfortunately, in the degraded climate of discussion that surrounds this issue, anti-MMR campaigners have a penchant for alleging conflicts of interest and corrupt influences on those who express support for MMR. So, if you can call it such, I declare this interest.

I have received no income in any form from any pharmaceutical or related company and I am not involved in any capacity in the litigation over MMR. Nor have I received any support from the Department of Health or any other government or academic agency. Indeed, the Department of Health refused to grant me study leave to write my last book and I did not request it for this one. Although I have already been accused of being a spokesman for the 'medical establishment', I have no links with any such institutions (beyond using their libraries).

*Michael Fitzpatrick*
*November 2003*

## Postscript

That MMR paper is the best example there has ever been of a very, very dodgy paper that has created a lot of discomfort and misery. (Dr Richard Smith, editor of the *British Medical Journal* quoted in the *Sunday Times*, 22 February 2004)

On 22 February 2004, in a major investigative feature in the *Sunday Times*, Brian Deer revealed that Dr Wakefield had failed to declare a conflict of interest in relation to the February 1998 *Lancet* paper in which he first alleged a link between MMR and autism (Deer, 2004a). Dr Wakefield had received £55,000 in Legal Aid funding to conduct investigations into children whose parents were seeking compensation from the manufacturers of MMR on the grounds that this vaccine had caused inflammatory bowel disease and autism. Dr Wakefield admitted that at least four of the twelve children included in the *Lancet* study were also involved in the investigations commissioned by Richard Barr, the solicitor leading the anti-MMR litigation (Wakefield, 2004). The Legal Aid funding was granted during the summer of 1996, with the specific objective of demonstrating a link between MMR and autism, at the same time that the children included in the *Lancet* study began to be investigated at the Royal Free Hospital[1]. Dr Wakefield did not inform either his colleagues at the Royal Free or Dr Richard Horton, the editor of *The Lancet*, about his links with the anti-MMR litigation and his personal interest in making the autism connection.

Dr Horton indicated that if he had been aware of Dr Wakefield's financial interest he would not have published his paper in *The Lancet* (Deer, 2004a). He described the paper as 'fatally' flawed and Dr Wakefield's denial that there was a conflict of interest as 'perverse'. Ten of Dr Wakefield's co-authors formally retracted the suggestion of a link between MMR and autism made in the 1998 paper (while insisting that the possibility of a distinctive gastrointestinal condition in children with autism merited further investigation) (Murch et al, 2004) (Dr John Linnell could not be contacted; Drs Wakefield and Harvey declined to sign). The Dublin-based virologist Professor John O'Leary, a close collaborator with Dr Wakefield (and who received £800,000 for his work for the anti-MMR litigation campaign) subsequently indicated that his investigations 'did not support the MMR–autism hypothesis' (Deer, 2004b). Using sophisticated molecular techniques, Professor O'Leary had sought – and failed – to identify fragments of measles virus in autistic children.

As a result of these revelations, Dr Wakefield has been referred to the General Medical Council (the doctors' disciplinary body) for further investigation. The Liberal Democrat MP Evan Harris has called for a judicial inquiry into the wider aspects of the case, including the role of the Legal Services Commission (formerly the Legal Aid Board) and the ethics of conducting invasive investigations into autistic children for the purposes of litigation or research, rather than according to clinical need.

The clues that Brian Deer investigated – the biased selection of cases in the *Lancet* study, the fact that it was Dr Wakefield alone who ensured that MMR was the focus of the paper (and the subsequent press conference) despite the lack of evidence – were already evident in 1998, long before the *Sunday Times* investigation: they are discussed in Chapters 7 and 8. The fact that, before Brian Deer, nobody bothered to pursue these clues does much to explain the impact of the MMR scare[2]. In a climate highly sensitive to health risks and increasingly distrustful of expert opinion, many – including prominent journalists and politicians – wanted to believe Dr Wakefield. Unfortunately, this meant that they suspended any critical or investigative instincts in relation to the campaign against MMR. As a result, one speculative paper, now repudiated by most of the team that produced it and by the editor who published it, has had the effect of reducing the uptake of MMR far below that required to maintain community resistance to measles, mumps and rubella.

Even after the *Sunday Times* revelations, journalists who had previously lauded Dr Wakefield as a courageous maverick were ready to justify his conduct and to present him as the victim of a smear campaign orchestrated by the government, the medical establishment and the drug companies (Phillips 2004, Caplin 2004, *Private Eye* 2004). The popular resonance for the MMR scare, and for conspiracy theories to explain why Dr Wakefield had become increasingly isolated and discredited, confirm that there are wider issues involved than Dr Wakefield's scientific or personal credibility. That is why this book seeks to place the (flawed) science of claims of a link between MMR and autism in the social and political context that allowed these claims to have such an impact on society.

*Michael Fitzpatrick*
*8 March 2004*

1   The Legal Services Commission received Dr Wakefield's application for funding on 6 June 1996; funds were released on 22 August. The children involved in the *Lancet* study were seen at the Royal Free between 25 July 1996 and 24 February 1997 (see *Sunday Times* 7 March 2004).
2   Brian Deer's earlier investigate work, in relation to the whooping cough vaccine scare, is discussed in Chapter 3.

## Acknowledgements

I am very grateful to my colleagues at Barton House Health Centre, who have had to endure discussions about MMR over lunch as well as during baby clinics and surgeries, especially to Matthew Bench our in-house immunisation and general child health expert. I also pay tribute to Mick Hume and all the staff at spiked-online.com – the Internet magazine that does not fear critical thinking – where many of the ideas in this book first appeared in article form.

I would also like to acknowledge helpful discussions with Helen Bedford, Virginia Bovell, Tracey Brown, Hilary Cass, Jenny Cunningham, Thomas Deichmann, Carole Dezateux, David Elliman, John Fitzpatrick, Fiona Fox, Frank Furedi, David Goldblatt, Paul Gringras, Martin Hewitt, Tom Jefferson, Gabriella Laing, Johnjoe McFadden, Elizabeth Mitchell, Simon March, Brent Taylor, David Thrower and Mark Wilks. Because most of these people will disagree with something in the book – and some with almost everything – I emphasise that they bear no responsibility for its contents.

My greatest debt is to my family: to my wife, Mary, a constant source of support and constructive criticism, and to my mother, Margaret, James' devoted grandma. I owe a special debt to my two sons, Michael and James, and this book is dedicated to them.

# 1

# INTRODUCTION: WHAT PARENTS NEED TO KNOW

By any rational standards of risk/benefit calculation, it is an illogical and potentially dangerous mistake for parents to be prepared to take their children in a car or in an aeroplane on holiday, but not to protect them with the MMR vaccine.

(Murch 2003 [Simon Murch was co-author of Dr Wakefield's 1998 *Lancet* paper])

## MMR is a good vaccine

In the public discussion following the London première of the anti-MMR television drama 'Hear the Silence' in September 2003 a journalist active in the campaign against MMR claimed that doctors had exaggerated the benefits of immunisation by failing to acknowledge that deaths from measles had been declining before MMR was introduced: 'Only 14 children' had died from measles in Britain in 1988 – the year MMR was launched. 'Only 14?' I exclaimed in horror (the number was in fact 18). This grotesque disregard for the loss of infant lives, not to mention the much higher toll of brain damage and respiratory disease, reveals the loss of moral bearings that afflicts anti-immunisation zealots. The fact that, after 18 deaths in one year, in the ten years following the introduction of MMR there were 'only' a handful of deaths from measles seems to me a powerful argument in favour of the vaccine.

The MMR vaccine is highly effective in preventing measles, mumps and rubella. Since its introduction in Britain, these once common diseases have become rare and a generation of children has been spared the illness, disability and death that these diseases can cause. In some countries, such as Finland, measles has been virtually eliminated (a few cases have been reported among newly arriving immigrants). In the USA, measles is now largely associated with imported cases (notably from Japan, where, for historical reasons, immunisation uptake is relatively low, and where around 100,000 cases every year cause between 50 and 100 deaths) (Noble, Miyasaka 2003). As a result of the anti-MMR campaign, the goal of measles eradication in Britain – within reach in the mid-1990s – is now unlikely to be achieved in the foreseeable future.

Although the mass immunisation campaign offers the prospect of ridding society of measles for good, the immediate benefit of MMR is to the individual child who receives it. Until measles and mumps have been eradicated, they are still a risk, albeit a small one, to every child. It is true that this risk is greatest to children who suffer from

*Table 1.1* Diseases that may return

| Diseases | Symptoms | Complications | Duration |
|----------|----------|---------------|----------|
| Measles | Fever, rash, cough, sore eyes, swollen glands, loss of appetite, unwell. | Ear infection: 1 in 20 Pneumonia/bronchitis: 1 in 25 Convulsion: 1 in 200 Diarrhoea: 1 in 6 Hospital admission: 1 in 100 Meningitis/encephalitis: 1 in 1,000 Subacute sclerosing panencephalitis (SSPE): 1 in 8,000 (under 2) Death: 1 in 2,500–5,000 | 5 days in bed; off school 10 days; adults longer. |
| Mumps | Painful, swollen glands, fever, headache, abdominal pain, loss of appetite, unwell. | Swollen testicles: 1 in 5 Meningitis/encephalitis: 1 in 200–5,000 Pancreatitis: 1 in 30 Deafness: 1 in 25 In pregnancy: miscarriage | 7–10 days |
| Rubella | Fever, headache, rash, sore eyes, throat, cough, swollen glands, joint pains, loss of appetite, unwell. | Joint symptoms Encephalitis: 1 in 6,000 Bleeding disorders: 1 in 3,000 In pregnancy: congenital rubella syndrome – deafness, blindness, heart problems, brain damage. | 48–72 hours |

*Table 1.2* MMR: much safer than the disease it prevents

| Condition | Rate after natural disease | Rate after MMR |
|---|---|---|
| Convulsions | 1 in 200 | 1 in 1,000 |
| Meningitis/encephalitis | 1 in 2,000–5,000 | 1 in 1,000,000 |
| Bleeding disorders | 1 in 3,000 | 1 in 100,000 |
| Severe allergic response | – | 1 in 100,000 |
| Deaths | 1 in 2,500–5,000 (depending on age) | 0 |

some condition causing diminished immunity, but it is also true that there is some risk even to healthy children. In recent epidemics in Italy, the Netherlands and Ireland around half of the fatalities from measles have occurred in children who were previously in good health. Mumps is less serious than measles but it is still an unpleasant disease with even more unpleasant complications (meningitis, deafness, sterility, pancreatitis). Rubella is a mild disease in children, but, if passed on to women during pregnancy, highly damaging to the developing fetus (causing mental handicap, deafness and visual impairment, heart defects and cerebral palsy). Since MMR, the congenital rubella syndrome has become rare.

The MMR vaccine is safe. In our risk-averse times it might be more fashionable to say that the risks associated with MMR are low or that the evidence that it causes serious adverse consequences (such as inflammatory bowel disease or autism) is weak. But when 500 million doses of a vaccine have been given in 80 countries over more than 30 years, and serious adverse reactions have been found to be extremely rare, then it is fair to describe it as 'safe'.

## Separate vaccines are a bad choice

Opting to give MMR as its three separate components makes no sense. Some campaigners blame the measles component of MMR for causing inflammatory bowel disease and autism. If they believe this, then why shouldn't the separate measles vaccine carry the same risks? Others believe that it is giving the combination of three vaccines in one go that causes damage to the infant immune system. But there is no evidence that this is the case and much evidence to the contrary (Offit 2002, Miller et al 2003).

Nor is there any scientific basis for leaving any particular interval between the three separate vaccines. In 1998 Dr Wakefield suggested twelve months; some clinics give them six months or six weeks apart.

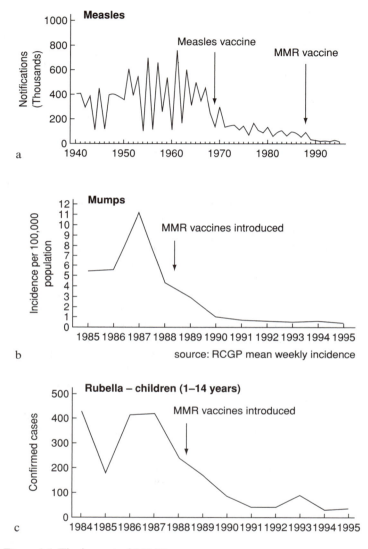

*Figure 1.1* The impact of MMR

At a public meeting at the Science Museum in London in January 2003, one paediatrician told of a private GP who had offered to give a child the three separate vaccines at the same time, to minimise the inconvenience to the parents. No country in the world offers separate vaccines as part of its childhood immunisation programme. No research has been carried out to explore the consequences of giving MMR in its separate components.

While the benefits of separate vaccines are nebulous, the dangers are clear. For however long the full programme of immunisations is delayed, the child is vulnerable to infection from the diseases protected against by the later immunisations. If children get one injection every 12 months from their first birthdays, they will be 3 before they are fully protected. If their parents also choose to give their 'pre-school booster' in three separate vaccines, they could be well on in junior school before the programme is finished. Six separate injections will be increasingly unpleasant for older children. It will also require at least one parent to take time out from work or other commitments to take children to clinics. Although parents committed to the campaign against MMR always insist that they would never miss a clinic appointment of such importance to their children, everybody else knows that some of these children are likely to miss out on some of the vaccines.

If parents choose to give their children MMR in the form of separate vaccines, this will certainly leave all these children unprotected for longer and will possibly leave some unprotected forever. This pool of unimmunised children creates the opportunity for outbreaks of measles (and mumps and rubella). When this happens, as we have seen, all children will be at risk, but the children who are most in danger are those who cannot be given live vaccines (because their immune system is suppressed by disease or medication), and babies in the first year of life. The risk to these children is high because they have no immunity to measles and measles is a highly infectious disease. If there is an epidemic such children are very likely to get measles and more likely than other children to get it in a more severe form, with a higher risk of short- and long-term complications. Campaigners against MMR and other vaccines sometimes ridicule the concept of 'herd immunity' because it implies treating human communities like those of farm animals. But for children with leukaemia or HIV, herd immunity is no joking matter: it may be the difference between life and death.

Campaigners often castigate the Department of Health for refusing to provide separate vaccines, claiming that when MMR was introduced this choice was denied (sometimes also claiming that it is still available in other countries). The facts are that when MMR was introduced the separate measles vaccine, which had been introduced 20 years earlier, was gradually phased out. Although the

5

rubella vaccine had previously been given to early teenage girls and, after childbirth, to women found not to be immune during pregnancy, a significant number of congenital rubella cases continued to occur. The strategy of including rubella in MMR given to infants aimed to reduce these numbers (and it has been successful in doing this). The mumps vaccine was not available as a separate vaccine before MMR. No country offers separate vaccines as an alternative to MMR (although in France the measles vaccine is still available to be given separately to babies attending nurseries before the age of 12 months, they are still recommended to have the MMR later).

It is the responsibility of the Department of Health to develop an immunisation programme that provides the best possible protection to children against a range of infectious diseases. It has to do this taking into account a wide range of factors, including the nature and risk of the diseases, and the efficacy and safety of the vaccines. These are complex matters and the programme is inevitably subject to change as research reveals unforeseen opportunities – or dangers – and new vaccines become available. The object of immunisation policy is not to provide a 'pick-and-mix' selection to the public, but to provide a coherent programme for the prevention of infectious diseases. This is one reason why, under the NHS, childhood immunisations have always been given free of charge. The danger of simply making vaccines available in the absence of an effective programme to ensure adequate uptake is illustrated by the experience in Greece where a poorly organised system of rubella vaccination resulted in an increased number of cases of the congenital syndrome (King 1999, Bedford, Elliman 2001: 116).

If the government were to offer separate vaccines as an alternative to MMR, it could be legitimately accused of putting political expediency before its responsibility to the health of children and to public health. No doubt the lawyers currently engaged in the anti-MMR cause would be ready to pursue litigation on these grounds when the inevitable consequences appeared in the form of children adversely affected by measles, mumps or rubella.

## MMR does not cause autism

Although it is not known what does cause autism, it is as clear as anything can be that MMR does not cause it. The theory that MMR causes autism is inconsistent with what is known about autism: its strongly genetic character, its association with a range of conditions that are present at birth and probably arise at an early stage of fetal development, and all the epidemiological data surveyed in Chapters 8 and 9. It is also inconsistent with the experience of MMR in Britain and in other countries: autism existed before MMR and, whatever the reason for the rise in the numbers of children diagnosed as autistic, this does not correlate with exposure to MMR. Furthermore, the proposed causal pathway through which MMR is supposed to result in autism is (as discussed in Chapter 9) highly speculative: not a single link in the complex chain of causality hypothesised by anti-MMR campaigners has been substantiated.

In response to the weight of evidence against their hypothesis, anti-MMR campaigners have scaled down their claims. Whereas they once claimed that MMR was to blame for an epidemic of autism, they now claim that it causes autism only in a small number of individuals who are rendered vulnerable by a range of other factors. Yet, more than five years after the MMR–autism hypothesis was first announced, its supporters have failed to demonstrate this link in a single child.

Under pressure from parents and their supporters who fervently believe in the MMR link, some authorities attempt to be conciliatory by conceding that, although scientific evidence does not support this in general, they 'cannot rule out' the possibility that it does cause autism in a small number of cases. But this is simply to assert the logical impossibility of proving a negative: that MMR can *never* cause autism. At a time when parents with children due for immunisation are being frightened off MMR by the autism scare, and when this scare is making autism parents feel guilty about having given their children MMR, conceding the logical impossibility of disproving the MMR–autism link in every single case is to use an abstract philosophical point to evade the real issue. The real issue is not whether the MMR–autism link can be disproved in every case, but whether it can be substantiated in any case. On this point the evidence provided by research conducted over the past five years, in a range of disciplines (notably virology and epidemiology) and in a number of countries, points overwhelmingly in the same direction: it fails to support the MMR–autism hypothesis. To continue to repeat in response to this body of evidence that 'we still cannot rule out the possibility of a link' is strictly true, but philosophically banal. Given the consequences for parents of the refusal to acknowledge the failure of exhaustive research to substantiate the MMR–autism hypothesis, persisting with this line is not only casuistry, but disingenuous.

## Autism is not about to be cured or defeated, but much can be done to help

Autists can learn some coping strategies, but their condition will never be 'cured'. And the rest of us must learn to stop wishing for a cure. Acceptance is all.

(Charlotte Moore, 'Mind the gap', *Guardian*, 23 April 2003)

The advances in the understanding of autism that have taken place over recent decades have not resulted in the development of any treatment that can alter the course of the condition in any fundamental way. Indeed the more precise identification of the genetic factors that predispose to autism and the clarification of the deficits in social interaction and communication have confirmed the profundity and complexity of the disorder and the extent of the resulting disability. In a sense these developments have emphasised the gulf between basic science and therapeutics, intensifying the distress and frustration of parents. Given the scale of the problems posed by autism and the current pace of scientific advance, it is highly unlikely that any cure will emerge within the lifetime of our children. 'Acceptance', as Charlotte Moore, mother of two autistic boys, writes, 'is all'. This does not mean adopting a fatalistic posture that nothing can be done, but it does mean parents accepting that the quest for a wonder cure is not likely to be helpful for their autistic child, for any other children they might have, or for themselves. Parents are entitled to feel sadness and anger when their child is diagnosed as autistic, but in time they need to stop railing at the world and direct their energies into strategies that will benefit their child and their families. Campaigns that channel parents' energies into the pursuit of wonder cures, or into futile confrontations with doctors, scientists and other professionals, or into litigation over vaccines, offer illusory hopes – and targets for blame and recrimination. At best they divert and dissipate already over-stretched parental energies; at worst they encourage an enduring rage that is likely to compound family difficulties, to intensify isolation and lead ultimately to demoralisation.

What works in autism? Early intervention with a programme such as the National Autistic Society's 'EarlyBird' scheme, which provides support and guidance for parents soon after their child has been diagnosed as autistic, is likely to benefit both child and parents. The programme, which includes training sessions and home visits, helps parents to understand their child's autism and shows them how to structure interaction in such a way as to encourage communication. It also suggests how to develop strategies to pre-empt problem behaviours and how to deal with those that occur. Organisers have a positive, practical approach: 'we do not offer a cure at EarlyBird, but we do offer hope'.

The consensus of a number of reviews of interventions is that methods based on procedures from special education and behavioural psychology are the best option for autistic children (Howlin 1998, Jordan et al 1998, 1999, New York State Department of Health 1999). These methods are used in a variety of structured approaches, such as the TEACCH programme developed by Schopler and Mesibov and colleagues in North Carolina. These programmes differ in theory, in technique and in level of intensity, but there is no evidence to confirm the superiority of any particular approach. The biggest problem facing children with autism and their parents is the grave shortage of places in schools with appropriate levels of resources and skills. The uneven and inadequate provision of respite care, to help the families of autistic children over weekends and holiday periods, is another serious problem.

Apart from behavioural methods, evidence is lacking for other forms of intervention, including 'physical' techniques (sensory integration, music therapy, auditory integration) and 'medical' treatments (hormonal, immunological, anti-yeast, vitamins and diets). There is some evidence to support a limited role for medication, such as the atypical antipsychotic drug risperidone, in the control of aggressive and self-injurious behaviour. For older, higher functioning, children there are a range of educational programmes, focusing in particular on social skills.

# 2

# THE MMR DEBACLE

BLAIR WARNING AS MEASLES PANIC GROWS

Faced with the lethal mix of tabloid uproar, mounting
parental anxiety and Conservative attempts to exploit
ministers' discomfort, Mr Blair denounced MMR critics
for scaremongering. 'The scaremongering – and it is scaremongering – about this vaccine is wrong. Often such scaremongering doesn't matter. In this case it does.'

(*Guardian*, 7 February 2002)

In February 2002 it was exactly four years since Dr Andrew
Wakefield published his article linking the MMR vaccine with
inflammatory bowel disease and autism (Wakefield et al 1998). In
the week preceding Mr Blair's statement, health officials had
responded to the MMR scare with a counter-scare: if parents were
worried about the dangers of MMR, outbreaks of measles in
Streatham, Gateshead and Teesside confirmed the risk to their children if they failed to get them immunised.

Ever since the 'Don't Die of Ignorance' campaign in 1987, and the
notorious 'tombstones and icebergs' advertising campaign, which
raised fears of the spread of AIDS in Britain out of all proportion
to the real risk, the government has used scares in the cause of health
promotion. Although Mr Blair says that such scaremongering 'often
doesn't matter', the MMR debacle confirms that it does. A decade of
health scares has contributed to a high level of public anxiety about
issues of health: any suggestion of a new risk is guaranteed a
panicky response, especially if it raises the possibility of a devastating disability afflicting healthy infants. This mood of anxiety is not
responsive to reassurance – and even less to counter-scares. As the
continuing decline in uptake of MMR has confirmed, both are likely
to be counterproductive. Scaremongering around MMR has made

parents fearful of having their children immunised and fearful of not having them immunised. Some opt one way or the other; many, understandably confused and bemused, put the decision off.

Eight months later, Mr Blair touched on another theme at the heart of the MMR controversy in his speech at the Labour Party conference in Blackpool (*The Times,* 2 October 2002). 'We've never been more individualist in our outlook', Mr Blair told delegates, even though globalisation and technological developments also cause 'massive insecurity'. He drew out the consequences of this intensely individualistic outlook in the spheres of health and education. Instead of the 'big state' and 'paternalistic welfare' 'that won't do today', 'people want an individual service for them'; they want 'personalised care, built around the individual patient or parent'. Mr Blair demanded change in the health service to 'put power in the hands of patients'.

But for four years anti-MMR campaigners had been asking the government to allow them to exercise their choice in favour of giving their children separate vaccines rather than the triple jab. Despite all Mr Blair's rhetoric about empowering individuals, the government had stuck doggedly to the line that medical experts had advised that the triple vaccine was best and that the choice of separate vaccines should not be made available. Indeed, the Department of Health took steps to restrict the availability of separate vaccines in Britain.

Some contradictions in New Labour policy as it impinges on MMR are readily apparent. The government is in favour of scaremongering in general, especially if it encourages the adoption of 'healthy lifestyles' or childhood immunisation. It is resolutely opposed to scaremongering when this raises public concerns about vaccine safety. The government is in favour of individual choice in general, but not when this means individual choice of separate vaccines. The MMR debacle is the story of the unfolding of these contradictions in the course of the 1990s.

## The rise of immunisation and the fall of MMR

In the early 1990s the programme of Mass Childhood Immunisation (MCI) in Britain was acclaimed as one of the great success stories of modern public health (Leese, Bosanquet 1992). A greater number of children were being immunised against a wider range of infectious diseases than ever before. Diseases that had caused devastating epidemics in living memory, and had produced a significant toll of death and disability into the post-war period, had virtually disappeared.

Immunisation was popular and widely credited with a decisive role in preventing disease. In 1992/93 the proportion of children immunised against diphtheria, tetanus and polio reached 95 per cent (an increase of more than 10 per cent over the previous decade) (DH 1997: 278). The uptake of the whooping cough jab, which had dropped below one third in the 1970s as a result of claims (subsequently discredited) that it caused brain damage, had climbed to 92 per cent in 1992 (see Chapter 3). Although improvements in living standards and public sanitation may have been the most important factors in the decline in infectious diseases in the past century, there can be little doubt that it was the MCI programme that ensured the virtual eradication of once lethal childhood diseases.

The introduction of the MMR immunisation in 1988 marks the high-tide of the MCI programme (Badenoch 1988). Although it offered protection against three diseases, this highly purified product contained little more than 10 per cent of the antigens (proteins and polysaccharides) contained in the old smallpox vaccination (Offit et al 2002). It offered a combination of high efficacy and a low incidence of adverse effects. Launched in 1988, its uptake passed 90 per cent within four years, and measles, the most serious of the three diseases, rapidly became a rarity. In the ten years before the first measles immunisation was introduced (in 1968) there were around 380,000 cases a year and 850 deaths (Bedford, Elliman 2001: 35). Between 1989 and 1998, there were four deaths associated with acute measles and 19 resulting from late complications.

'One more push' was the central theme of vaccination policy in the early 1990s, as health authorities and health professionals joined in a concerted effort to achieve the target of 95 per cent uptake of MMR required to guarantee 'herd immunity' (Nicoll et al 1989, Leese, Bosanquet 1992, Egan et al 1994). (When vaccine levels are at a high level in a community, the risk of disease is so low that even those who are not immune are unlikely to be affected. Achieving this level of 'herd immunity' is of critical importance in protecting children who are suffering from leukaemia or some other form of immune deficiency and therefore cannot receive live vaccines such as MMR and polio.) Discussion centred around the problems of organising baby clinics and GP surgeries to reach a residual group of socially disadvantaged children whose parents tended to neglect to get them immunised. Although anti-immunisation campaigns stretching back to the nineteenth century continued to attract devotees of homeopathy and other modes of alternative health, they remained a feeble force against the powerful consensus in support of immunisation (Wolfe, Sharp 2002).

Then disaster struck the MMR. In February 1998 Dr Andrew Wakefield and his colleagues at the Royal Free Hospital in North London published a paper in *The Lancet* postulating a link between MMR, and autism (Wakefield et al 1998). By 2002 national uptake of MMR, far from reaching 95 per cent, had fallen below 85 per cent; in some areas, notably in inner London, it was below 75 per cent (Government Statistical Service, September 2002). It is true that the fall was much less precipitous than that of the whooping cough immunisation 20 years earlier, but it still means that, instead of disappearing, cases of measles, mumps and rubella, with all their grim complications, are likely to return.

What went wrong? How could one paper do such damage to a well-established immunisation programme? How did an anti-immunisation outlook that was marginal a decade earlier suddenly become a mainstream influence? Why were attempts to bolster confidence in the MMR so ineffective? These are the questions at the heart of the MMR debacle.

Uptake of MMR did not simply collapse after February 1998: the pattern of its decline, *before* as well as after that date suggests that the Wakefield paper was not the only factor. In the mid-1990s, before the MMR–autism link had been suggested, there were already signs that MMR was in trouble. The level of uptake, which had risen steadily up to 1992, reached a plateau at around 92 per cent, at which

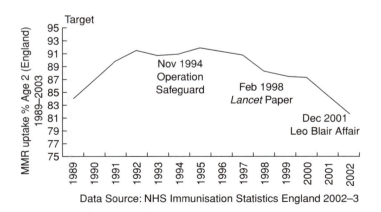

Data Source: NHS Immunisation Statistics England 2002–3

*Figure 2.1* The rise and decline of MMR

13

it remained for the next five years. In 1997, uptake declined for the first time, by about 1 per cent. This followed the adverse publicity for the immunisation programme resulting from Operation Safeguard in November 1994, when schoolchildren received a special measles and rubella (MR) immunisation. It also followed publicity in 1995 for Dr Wakefield's early work suggesting a link between measles or measles vaccination and inflammatory bowel diseases (Roberts 1995). In 1998, the year in which the MMR–autism scare erupted, uptake fell by a further 2 per cent. However, over the next two years, uptake stabilised, perhaps indicating the limited impact of the scare, the effectiveness of official reassurances or simply the resilience of the MCI programme. Then, in 2001/02, as MMR attracted more frequent publicity in a wider range of newspapers and became the focus of political controversy (notably over whether the infant Leo Blair had received his MMR and the demand for single vaccines), uptake fell by 4 per cent.

In examining more closely these different stages in the decline of MMR, we necessarily focus on the particularities of the immunisation controversy. It is however important to recognise the influence of wider factors on parents' attitudes and decisions in relation to MMR. For example, commentators frequently draw attention to the impact of the BSE/CJD scandal in undermining public confidence in both scientific expertise and government reassurances. Yet, as we have seen, uptake of MMR was stagnant for four years before the 'mad cow disease' scare erupted in March 1996; it did not fall substantially until two years later. Although the publication of the MMR–autism link did hit uptake, it declined more sharply three years later as the controversy widened (despite the continuing lack of evidence for the link). The 1990s was a decade in which anxieties about health were reflected in the impact of a wide range of health scares and environmental alarums (Fitzpatrick 2001). A heightened sense of individual insecurity was expressed in a popular mood of risk aversion and a culture of litigation (Furedi 2002). The narrowing scope of the realm of politics encouraged the politicisation of issues of health and disease, family relationships and childrearing practices. All these factors had a significant and growing impact on the MMR controversy throughout the 1990s.

## Before the storm

In the early 1990s, discussions in health policy circles about how to improve vaccine uptake distinguished two groups of parents whose children were not being immunised. These can be broadly categorised as 'passive defaulters' and 'active resisters'.

Passive defaulters were characteristically low-income families experiencing various forms of deprivation and social exclusion (Egan et al 1994). Some were homeless or Travellers. Their failure to have their children immunised was partly attributed to 'parental reluctance' and partly to 'professional apathy', to the poor provision of primary care and child health services, notably in inner-city areas. Measures to reach this group, both with health education initiatives and with measures to improve the training, motivation and organisation of local health service staff, were the central themes of official policy.

The active resisters were middle-class, well-educated parents who had chosen not to have their children immunised. This group formed the focus of a qualitative sociological study by Anne Rogers and David Pilgrim, who, between December 1992 and March 1993, interviewed 19 mothers who had refused to have their children immunised (Rogers, Pilgrim 1994). Given that this group may be regarded as representative of the subsequent wave of MMR refusers, it is worth looking at the results of this fascinating study more closely. A number of themes emerged.

First, parents were concerned about the risks of adverse consequences of immunisation, which they felt had been played down in the official information. These fears drew attention to the paradox that, as the risk of the diseases that immunisation protected against became more remote (and folk memories of these diseases faded), the risk to any individual child of adverse effects tended relatively to increase and certainly came to loom larger in parental concerns.

Second, these parents expressed sceptical views towards 'biomedicine' and an openness to alternatives, particularly homeopathy. Holistic and homeopathic concepts were a significant influence on their resistance to immunisation, which was regarded as potentially damaging to the immune system and to babies' naturally acquired immunity.

Third, they were suspicious of the apparent convergence of interests among the medical profession, the government and the vaccine manufacturers in the promotion of the MCI programme. The financial incentive for GPs to meet immunisation targets 'was a repetitive theme in interviews'; the launch of MMR was regarded as 'a marketing strategy for financial gain'. (The authors note that the question of financial interest was not raised in parents' accounts of their relations with homeopathic and alternative practitioners, even though these practitioners were entirely reliant on private fees.)

Rogers and Pilgrim commented on the trend for anti-immunisation attitudes to evolve over time: for example, some mothers who had agreed to the immunisation of older children, balked at immunising their new babies. This consolidation appeared to take place partly as a result of further reading and reflection and partly in response to negative experiences with doctors and other health professionals. The authors also noted the growing cohesion of anti-immunisation views as a result of a number of homeopathic publications and also of the emergence in the early 1990s of new campaign groups such as 'The Informed Parent' and the 'What Doctors Don't Tell You' bulletins (subsequently gathered together in the *Vaccination Bible*) (see Chaitow 1987, McTaggart 1996, 2000).

In a more substantial reflection upon the results of their study, Rogers and Pilgrim noted the increasingly acrimonious confrontation between self-righteous medical 'zealots' promoting immunisation, and 'dissenting parents', who, 'with their mixture of cynicism about bio-medicine and anger about their rights as citizen consumers, exude their own version of outrage and indignation' (Rogers, Pilgrim 1995: 87). One of the ironies revealed by this study was that the 'active resisters' tended to accept the principles of a healthy lifestyle – as recommended by the government – in matters such as diet and exercise, smoking and drinking alcohol. Only when it came to immunisation did they reject official health promotion propaganda, sometimes expressing the conviction that their virtuous lifestyle – further manifested in prolonged breastfeeding and conscientious childcare – provided their children with adequate protection against infectious diseases.

In a policy discussion published alongside the Rogers and Pilgrim study in a Health Education Authority pamphlet, supporters of the immunisation programme noted the 'lack of suitable educational materials' for 'non-consenting parents' (Egan et al 1994). They recommended something that put the case in favour of vaccines 'in a scientifically readable way, without the use of fear arousal techniques'. Unfortunately, it was another five years before such material became readily available (Elliman, Bedford 1999, 2001). In the meantime, whether or not official efforts focusing on passive defaulters had any positive effect on this group, they were likely to be counterproductive for active resisters. The Rogers and Pilgrim study revealed these parents' contempt for information provided by health promotion sources, which they regarded as inadequate, emotionally exploitative and as 'state propaganda'. Furthermore, the continuation of the incentive scheme for GPs – which undoubtedly contributed to improved uptake among passive defaulters in inner-city areas – intensified the cynicism of the active resisters.

There can be little doubt that Rogers and Pilgrim's terse 1995 judgement – that 'currently, MCI is hegemonic' – was accurate (Rogers, Pilgrim 1995: 87). A possible explanation for the steady level of uptake is that any success vaccine promotion might have had among the passive defaulters was balanced by a growing number of active resisters. Yet, overall, public confidence in MMR remained high. When two brands of MMR vaccine were withdrawn in 1992 following a number of cases of aseptic meningitis caused by the particular strain of the mumps vaccine component, this attracted virtually no public controversy and had a negligible impact on uptake. (The case of the Urabe mumps strain has since become a recurrent theme of the anti-MMR campaign; see Chapter 8.) However, Rogers and Pilgrim had identified the growing influence of the individualistic outlook championed by Tony Blair in his Blackpool speech a decade later. This was expressed in a growing hostility to immunisation among a small but significant section of the population. This led them to conclude that the hegemony of MCI was 'precarious and time-limited':

> In advanced Western capitalist societies, increasing expectations of consumer rights in service transactions have led to the need for greater availability of information and the citizen's right to accept or reject a product. The MCI programme fits poorly with these expectations, leading to a conflict of values and interests between state/medical paternalism and citizen consumerism.
>
> (Rogers, Pilgrim 1995: 88)

As the MMR debacle unfolded, this was to prove a highly prescient warning.

# 3

# TROUBLE WITH VACCINATIONS

The following are comments made at the February 1998 press conference at the Royal Free Hospital in London at which Dr Wakefield's *Lancet* paper suggesting a link between MMR and autism was launched:

> 'There is sufficient concern in my own mind for a case to be made for vaccines to be given individually at not less than one year intervals.'
>
> (Dr Andrew Wakefield)

> 'Measles vaccines are among the safest and most effective vaccines ever developed.'
>
> (Professor Arie Zuckerman, Dean of
> Royal Free Medical School)

> 'This link is unproven and measles is a killing infection. If this precipitates a scare and immunisation rates go down, as sure as night follows day, measles will return and children will die.'
>
> (Dr Simon Murch, paediatric gastroenterologist
> and co-signatory of the *Lancet* paper)

Shortly before Christmas 2002, our practice nurse asked me to have a look at a 14-year-old boy with a rash: 'I think he might have measles'. Sure enough he had the typical red blotchy patches, the fever, the harsh cough, the sore red eyes. He even had the tiny mouth ulcers, known as Koplik's spots, that, as medical students, we were always told to look out for but never seemed to find. Most strikingly, he was quite ill: his red face and streaming eyes were a vivid reminder of the sheer misery of measles. Saliva tests confirmed the diagnosis. We asked if he minded if some of our colleagues had a glimpse of his rash. Most doctors and nurses under the age of 50 have never seen a case of measles, so this was an opportunity not to be missed. This boy was a Polish Gypsy, recently arrived in London, who had not been vaccinated as an infant. (This is unusual in this community whose members, perhaps having a greater respect for the dangers of infectious disease than is now common in Britain, are notably conscientious in getting their children immunised.) Fortunately, this outbreak did not extend beyond a handful of family members and our patient made a fairly rapid recovery.

Being over the threshold of middle age, I have a better memory of measles than is now widespread either among doctors or in the general public. As a medical student in the mid-1970s, I spent a couple of months in a mission hospital in Tanzania where I saw children dying at an alarming rate from measles. The racking cough, the sunken, inflamed eyes and the peeling skin were unforgettable features of this devastating infection. As a junior hospital doctor in Britain in the early 1980s, I recall admitting a child with a high fever one night for observation, only for the telltale rash to appear the next day. It was not so unusual to see children being nursed in darkened rooms – to ease the sore eyes of measles – and under a red blanket – a traditional measure for 'bringing out the rash'. When I started as a trainee GP in East London, cases of measles were fairly common. My trainer always insisted that I prescribe antibiotics to forestall the dangers of secondary ear and chest infections, a counsel based on long experience of these complications rather than on strict observance of microbiological guidelines. He was also keen to ensure that I completed the appropriate 'notification of infectious disease' form, perhaps as much because it attracted a small fee as out of a concern to keep the public health authorities informed about the progress of any epidemic.

In more recent years, parents have sometimes brought children into the surgery, declaring 'I think she's got measles', but one glance at their healthy-looking and cheerful toddler playing in the corner – despite a bit of a cough, a few snuffles and some pale spots on the trunk – is enough to make this diagnosis highly improbable. It also prompts the reflection that these parents have obviously never seen a child with measles, and this is increasingly true of grandparents too.

Once reassured that their child probably has one of hundreds of viruses that cause minor coughs and colds and vague rashes, working parents' main concern is 'how long is this likely to last?' The answer is 'perhaps a few days'. If the diagnosis was measles, the answer would be 'two weeks, if you're lucky'. It would also mean two weeks of unremitting toil, caring for an often-inconsolable toddler who is likely to demand attention day and night for the duration of the illness. It is not widely recognised that the sort of childcare arrangements that allow both parents of young children to go out to work have been made possible in part by the virtual eradication of once common childhood diseases like measles. Today's parents do not expect to have to spend weeks caring for sick children in a way that was commonplace only a generation ago. Nor are grandparents or other extended family members so readily available for nursing duties.

Mumps is another almost-forgotten illness. Yet I remember looking after a child with mumps meningitis in hospital (until around 15 years ago mumps was one of the most common causes of admission with meningitis). Now we rarely see the hamster-shaped jaw-line, with bulging parotid glands pushing out the ears, that was once the familiar sign of mumps. Although it was never easy to be sure about the rash of rubella, its impact on the unborn babies of pregnant women can be devastating. In the 1960s there was an outbreak of rubella in London among newly arrived immigrants from the Caribbean: I have two patients who, as a result, were born with the multiple severe mental and physical handicaps of the congenital rubella syndrome.

Doctors remember the infectious diseases of childhood differently from other people. Some of my friends and patients nostalgically recall spending happy days off school with mothers and grand-mothers. No doubt for most people these illnesses were not so severe; for others, a benign amnesia seems to have blanked out the distressing aspects of the experience, as it often does the pains of childbirth. In the nature of their work, doctors' attention is drawn to the more severe cases and to patients who experience complications, most of all to the occasional fatalities, and these linger long in the memory. Talking over today's vaccination controversies with a now-elderly, long-retired paediatrician, he recalled seeing children with polio in the 1950s being kept alive with primitive 'iron lung' ventilators. He was horrified that the achievements of mass childhood immunisation were now questioned and at the prospect that diseases he had seen vanquished might return.

## Anti-vaccination campaigns past and present

To grasp the current predicament of immunisation policy, we need to put the MMR controversy into a wider context. When current concerns about MMR erupted in the late 1990s, some commentators drew parallels with the influence of anti-vaccination campaigns of the past, notably that against smallpox in the nineteenth century and against whooping cough in the 1970s. Supporters of the immunisation programme often illustrate their talks and articles with anti-vaccination cartoons from the nineteenth century, suggesting that these campaigns and their associated prejudices are always with us, but merely fluctuate in intensity over the years.

In a widely quoted article, Robert Wolfe and Lisa Sharp argue that 'the activities of today's propagandists against immunisation are directly descended from, indeed little changed from, those of the anti-vaccinationists of the late nineteenth century' (Wolfe, Sharp 2002: 430). The authors provide a table of quotations from each era, under the heading 'Anti-vaccination arguments, past and present'. The parallels are indeed striking: vaccines are blamed for a wide range of disorders (whose causes are otherwise unknown); doctors and vaccine manufacturers are in an 'unholy alliance for profit'; vaccines are 'poisonous chemical cocktails'; there has been a 'cover-up' of the adverse effects of vaccines; vaccine programmes mark a step 'towards totalitarianism'; vaccines are either ineffective or provide only temporary immunity; a healthy lifestyle provides a better protection against infectious diseases. The 'uncanny similarities' in these arguments suggest, according to the authors, 'an unbroken transmission of core beliefs and attitudes over time'.

Yet, historical accounts of anti-vaccination campaigns reveal more discontinuity than continuity. Vaccination against smallpox – a cause of devastating epidemics in nineteenth century Britain – was made compulsory by the Vaccination Act of 1853. Although there was little attempt at enforcement in the early years, after the Europe-wide epidemic of 1870/71, the authorities began to prosecute defaulters. In Leicester, for example, there were more than 6,000 prosecutions between 1869 and 1881 (Killick Millard 1948, Swales 1992). Some 64 people were imprisoned and 193 suffered 'distraint upon goods', 'the latter' according to one account, 'often being effected with much difficulty owing to popular sympathy with the defendants'. Such incidents provoked widespread support for anti-vaccination leagues in Britain, continental Europe and North America. An anti-vaccination demonstration in Leicester in 1885

21

claimed an attendance of 100,000. Continuing agitation in Britain led to the establishment of a Royal Commission, which reported in 1896, upholding vaccination but recommending the abolition of cumulative penalties against defaulters. A new Vaccination Act in 1898 duly abolished such penalties and introduced a clause allowing parents who did not believe that vaccination was efficacious or safe to obtain a certificate of exemption on grounds of conscience. Although this effectively marked the end of coercion and of mass anti-vaccination campaigning, it was not until 1948 that compulsory vaccination was finally abandoned.

What is striking in the post-war years, during which new immunisations were introduced and uptake steadily increased, is that anti-vaccination campaigns, if they existed at all, had negligible influence. Even in the 1980s, when immunisation uptake increased rapidly, and when alternative health practices such as homeopathy began to gain in popularity, anti-vaccination ideas remained marginal. The strength of the medical consensus in favour of immunisation was such that the society of medically qualified homeopaths formally endorsed this allopathic intervention, which was considered anathema by traditional homeopaths (Bedford, Elliman 2001: 59). It was not until the late 1980s and early 1990s that anti-immunisation sentiment re-emerged and spread rapidly from a small number of people influenced by alternative health beliefs to find a much wider resonance in British society. The explanation for this phenomenon must be sought, not in the timeless appeal of superficially similar anti-immunisation arguments, but in the specific circumstances of modern Britain.

An apparent exception to this argument is the campaign against the whooping cough (pertussis) vaccine in the mid-1970s. This scare had no direct connection with the earlier anti-vaccination campaigns: it arose in response to a report by a senior medical figure of specific adverse effects of the vaccine and this remained the sole concern of parents who refused to have their children immunised. It did not provoke a wider questioning of the principles of immunisation or the conduct of the immunisation programme. Although the whooping cough vaccine scare had little in common with the anti-smallpox vaccine campaigns of the nineteenth century, it is often cited as the forerunner of the current anti-MMR campaign (indeed, as a link in the seamless progress of anti-vaccinationism through the ages) (Baker 2003). The title of an editorial in the *British Medical Journal* summed up this view: 'MMR vaccination and autism 1998: Déjà vu – pertussis and brain damage 1974?' (Nicoll et al, 1998). A closer look at the whooping cough vaccine scare reveals striking similarities with the MMR controversy, but also crucial differences that illuminate the specific character of the current crisis.

## MMR: Déjà vu?

In March 1974 consultant paediatric neurologist Dr John Wilson published a study of 36 cases of children who had been admitted to Great Ormond Street Children's Hospital in London, over a period of 11 years, with 'neurological complications' following immunisation against whooping cough (pertussis) (Kulenkampff, Schwartzman, Wilson 1974).

The children who had been admitted to hospital had usually received their vaccination against whooping cough in the combined form of the triple vaccination against diphtheria, tetanus and pertussis (DTP). Although Dr Wilson insisted that his conclusions were 'tentative' and his study merely 'hypothesis-generating', it was widely interpreted as demonstrating that whooping cough immunisation caused brain damage. Dr Wilson and a small body of vocal supporters – most notably Glasgow community medicine professor Gordon Stewart – launched a campaign against the whooping cough vaccine. The scare was taken up on television and in the newspapers and made a major public impact. An Association of Parents of Vaccine-Damaged Children was formed and some 200 families were soon pursuing compensation claims against vaccine manufacturers, the government and family GPs. By 1976, vaccine uptake had dropped from 80 per cent to 30 per cent[1].

The campaign against the whooping cough vaccine appeared to be at least partially vindicated by the publication in 1981 of the preliminary results of the National Childhood Encephalopathy Study (Miller et al 1981). This had been set up in 1976 in response to the early reports of adverse reactions to the vaccine and included all young children admitted to hospital with severe acute neurological illnesses that could in any way be attributable to whooping cough immunisation. This preliminary report concluded that the whooping

---

1    The following account is based on reports in the medical journals, the judgment of Lord Justice Stuart-Smith in *Loveday* v *Renton and Another* (Queen's Bench Division, *The Times* 31 March 1988, No 1982 L 1812, (Transcript: Chilton Vint) and Brian Deer's excellent retrospective investigation (Deer 1998). Gangarosa et al (1998) provide a review of the impact of anti-vaccine movements on whooping cough internationally.

cough had, in a small number of cases, caused permanent brain damage: it estimated a risk of 1 in 310,000 – a figure that was accepted, and widely quoted, by vaccination authorities in Britain and around the world. Here matters stood until the claims for compensation came to court.

The first test case, that of Johnnie Kinnear born in 1969, reached court in 1986 but ended abruptly when it became clear that his mother had lied about the date of onset of his symptoms (Deer 1998). When the next case, that of Susan Loveday, born in 1970, came before Lord Justice Stuart-Smith in the spring of 1988, he insisted on first clarifying the question of whether whooping cough vaccine could cause brain damage. (Given the shift of concern towards autism as the specific disorder attributed to the MMR vaccine, it is interesting to note that, whereas in most of the cases blamed on the whooping cough vaccine the child suffered from epileptic fits, Susan Loveday was said to be autistic [Deer 1998: 50].)

In a trial lasting four months, the court heard 19 expert witnesses as Stuart-Smith LJ subjected the case against whooping cough vaccine to the most rigorous scrutiny: his judgment ran to 100,000 words and took two days to read (Bowie 1990). After insisting on reviewing the raw data of the National Childhood Encephalopathy Survey, Stuart-Smith LJ exposed a range of biases and errors that resulted in the conclusion of the preliminary report that the vaccine (rarely) caused brain damage. He found 'no evidence of permanent brain damage' and concluded that the widely quoted risk of 1 in 310,000, 'cannot be supported' and that 'any substituted figure would be so enormous as to be meaningless'. He also found that there was no conclusive evidence supporting any of the proposed mechanisms through which the vaccine was supposed to cause brain damage.

The judgment was highly critical of Dr Wilson (he was 'so completely committed to the view that the vaccine could cause brain damage that he was reluctant to re-examine evidence') and of other expert witnesses supporting the plaintiff's case against the vaccine. (A review of Wilson's original 36 cases revealed that in only 12 was there a close temporal association between the vaccine and manifestations of brain damage – most commonly epileptic fits. In the notorious case of twin girls, who were included in the 36 but had subsequently died of a rare genetic disorder, it was discovered that they had never received the whooping cough vaccine.) Noting the persistent tendency of critics of the vaccine to present the temporal association of vaccination and neurological events as evidence of causation, he quoted Dr Johnson: 'It is incident I am afraid, in physicians above all men, to mistake subsequences for consequences'.

This is how Stuart-Smith LJ concluded his classic judgment:

> When I embarked on consideration of the preliminary issue, I was impressed by the case reports and what was evidently a widely held belief that the vaccine could, albeit rarely, cause permanent brain damage. I was ready to accept that this belief was well founded. But over the weeks that I have listened to and examined the evidence and arguments I have become more and more doubtful that this is so. I have now come to the clear conclusion that the Plaintiff fails to satisfy me on the balance of probability that pertussis vaccine can cause permanent brain damage in young children. It is possible that it does; the contrary cannot be proved. But in the result the Plaintiff's claim must fall.

Subsequent follow-up reports on the cases included in the National Childhood Encephalopathy Study and authoritative reviews have provided further epidemiological support for this legal judgment (Miller et al 1993, Golden 1990).

While controversy raged over the vaccine, whooping cough returned: epidemics between 1977 and 1979 resulted in 27 deaths and 17 cases of permanent brain damage. While there was disagreement over whether the vaccine caused brain damage rarely or not at all, there could be no dispute that whooping cough caused both damage and death on a substantial scale (Preston 1980, Golden 1990). By

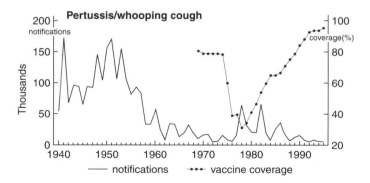

*Figure 3.1* The impact of the whooping cough vaccine scare

1988, the total number of deaths resulting from more than 300,000 notified cases of whooping cough was estimated as 'at least 70' (Nicoll et al 1998).

There are striking parallels between the whooping cough and MMR scares. Both emerged from studies presenting a small series of case reports. Both put great emphasis on the close temporal association between vaccination and the appearance of the adverse effect. Defenders of the vaccines pointed out that both fits and autism commonly appeared around the time of immunisation and that, if one followed the other, coincidence was the most likely explanation. Although readily criticised for being open to bias in their selection of cases, and for confusing association with causation, case report studies had a profound effect on public opinion, particularly when presented in the form of 'human interest' stories in the popular media.

Another common feature of both anti-vaccine campaigns was their difficulty in explaining how the vaccine produced the adverse effect with which it was associated. It is interesting to note that although some two decades separated the campaigns, they put forward strikingly similar theories. Some critics proposed that the vaccine produced a neurotoxic effect (via effects on adenosine/glutamate neurotransmitters in the case of whooping cough vaccine, via opioid peptides in the case of MMR). Others argued for an auto-immune process (an adjuvant effect of immunisation in enhancing the immune response to viral antigens in the case of whooping cough vaccine; an anti-myelin antibody response with MMR). The speculative character of these explanations encouraged some to combine these and other theories into increasingly complex (and increasingly unsatisfactory) 'multifactorial' explanations.

As evidence mounted against the anti-vaccinationists in both campaigns, they tended to retreat from claiming that adverse reactions were a common cause of serious disorders, to arguing that they did so only in small numbers of children, in whom there was some inherent, probably genetic, susceptibility. Leading proponents of the case against vaccines had another common fallback position: what Dr Wilson termed 'double reaction' cases and Dr Wakefield called 're-challenge' or 'double hit' cases. In these cases adverse reactions, or increasingly severe reactions, were noted after two or more exposures to the vaccine (whooping cough vaccine is routinely administered in a schedule of three immunisations in the first year; MMR is administered at around 15 months and again in the form of a 'pre-school booster'). There was, however, no better explanation for double- than single-dose vaccine effects.

Perhaps the most striking difference between the whooping cough vaccine and the MMR vaccine scares is their differential impact. Whereas uptake of whooping cough vaccine dropped precipitously to 30 per cent, MMR fell by only 7 per cent from a much higher baseline level in the four years after the publication of the Wakefield paper (from 92 to 85 per cent). The resilience of MMR vaccination is all the more surprising given the wider political impact of the Wakefield campaign compared with that of Wilson and Stewart. Although the whooping cough scare produced a dramatic fall in vaccine uptake, it did not become a major political issue. By contrast the MMR scare, though causing a much smaller drop in uptake, created a major stir in British politics.

The differing impact of these two scares reflects the changing character of British society over the past quarter of a century. In the mid-1970s parental (usually maternal) decisions about immunisation were largely private and personal, influenced more by immediate family members than by either health professionals or the wider debate. These decisions had an instinctive and pragmatic character; they were rarely based on any familiarity with the medical or scientific literature. Parents did not turn up at baby clinics in those days armed with anti-vaccination pamphlets and documents downloaded from the Internet.

By contrast, in the late 1990s parental discussions were both intensely personal (tending to involve fathers as well as mothers) and subject to wider public and political influences. Decisions about MMR have tended to reflect attitudes on the range of issues raised by the controversy: the authority of medical science and the medical profession, and the trustworthiness of vaccine manufacturers, civil servants and politicians. Whatever parents' decision on MMR, the issue of vaccination was a focus of considerable parental anxiety as discussion, and sometimes argument, raged among family and friends. The inclination of some parents to delay vaccination in the hope that matters would become clearer tended only to prolong the agony. The intensive media coverage of the issue and the involvement of politicians both reflected and encouraged this high level of popular concern about MMR. Thus, although uptake of MMR did not fall as dramatically as that of the whooping cough vaccine, it is arguable that the scare has had a more profound impact on society. The controversy around the demand for separate vaccines illustrates the wider political consequences of the MMR scare.

## The separate vaccines campaign

Dr Wakefield first suggested that parents should give the MMR in its three separate components at intervals of 12 months at the press conference launching his *Lancet* paper in February 1998 (*Guardian*, 27 February 1998). However, demand for separate vaccines grew slowly over the next three years. It increased in December 2000 when the Conservative MP Julie Kirkbride announced her intention to introduce a Vaccination of Children (Parental Choice) Bill the following year. Although, as a private member's Bill, this stood little chance of being enacted, its main purpose was to promote the anti-MMR campaign. Mrs Kirkbride, already a celebrity political parent (her husband is also a Conservative MP), was duly photographed with her children who were to receive separate vaccines – from the private GP Peter Mansfield, who was subsequently summoned to appear before the General Medical Council to explain his defiance of medical orthodoxy. This incident (which culminated in his exoneration in December 2001 when the GMC wisely refused to discipline him) served only to publicise the separate vaccine issue further.

It was another intervention 12 months later by Mrs Kirkbride that gave the separate vaccine campaign and the wider MMR–autism controversy its biggest boost. On 19 December 2001, during Prime Minister's Questions in the House of Commons, she inquired of Tony Blair whether his infant son Leo had received his MMR vaccination. Mr Blair's equivocal response was probably the most significant public relations setback for MMR since Dr Wakefield's initial allegations. Although he refused to disclose whether Leo had been immunised (claiming that this was a private family matter), Mr Blair indicated his support for the official line on MMR. While loyal supporters defended the Blairs' claim to privacy, other ministers (such as Yvette Cooper) disclosed their decision to give their children MMR. Critics insisted that immunisation was a matter of public health, not personal treatment, and recalled the willingness of members of the Royal Family to disclose that they had given their children the whooping cough vaccine following the 1970s scare. To the public, Mr Blair's stand seemed disingenuous: few doubted that if Leo had been immunised his parents would have been happy to publicise the fact. Given Cherie Blair's well-known proclivity for New Age charms and alternative healthcare, many believed that she had opted against MMR. The consequences for the public reputation of MMR were grim: if the Prime Minister's family doubted its safety, why should the public trust it?

Mr Blair's continuing evasiveness on MMR ensured that the controversy rumbled on into the New Year. The MMR–autism link was no longer a debate among medical experts, or even among specialist journalists and campaigning parents; now it became an issue for politicians, for political columnists and for leader-writers. In February, Dr Liam Fox, Shadow Health Minister and himself a GP, came out in support of the demand for separate vaccines, and the whole issue increasingly assumed a party-political form. At the opposite end of the political spectrum, the Scottish Socialist Party took the same line. The Liberal Democrats faced both ways: health spokesman Dr Evan Harris opposed calls for separate vaccines, while some parliamentary colleagues, such as Nick Harvey, upheld parents' rights to opt for separate vaccines in preference to their children having no vaccination at all. The MMR controversy has produced an unprecedented breakdown in the long-established cross-party consensus on vaccination policy. Party-political divisions were reflected in the press: the *Daily Mail*, *The Sun* and the *Daily Telegraph* supported the anti-MMR campaign; the *Mirror* and *The Express* were more sympathetic to the government line.

The Prime Minister and his medical advisers became increasingly defensive and began to sound petulant. While Mr Blair accused his critics of scaremongering, Chief Medical Officer Liam Donaldson declared that if the government were to approve separate vaccines it would be 'playing Russian roulette' with children's lives. This was a most inept metaphor: whatever he meant by it, it was widely interpreted as an accusation that *parents* were behaving irresponsibly towards their children by giving them separate vaccines.

The key problem was that New Labour's stand against separate vaccines ran counter to one of its central policy themes: the empowerment of the individual consumer, particularly in public services. This point was well made by the National Autistic Society in its March 2002 'position statement':

> The Government promotes choice in many areas of public policy. In rejecting it here it may fail to recognise assertions of patients' autonomy and a perception of paternalism may well have caused some of the reluctance to vaccinate.
>
> (NAS March 2002)

In January 2001, in the same week that Dr Wakefield held a press conference questioning the safety of MMR (see Chapter 8), Sir Donald Irvine, outgoing President of the General Medical Council gave a lecture at the Royal Society of Medicine. He used the occasion to reiterate the central theme of his drive to reform and modernise the medical profession:

> The cultural flaws in the medical profession show up as excessive paternalism, lack of respect for patients and their right to make decisions about their care, secrecy and complacency about poor practice.
>
> (*Guardian*, 16 January 2001)

Criticisms of doctors for being aloof and arrogant, authoritarian and paternalistic were recurrent themes of inquiries into scandals such as that over retained organs at Alder Hey Hospital and the children's heart surgery unit at Bristol (both of which reported in 2001, having a major public impact). Reformers, such as Dr Irvine and Professor Ian Kennedy who presided over the Bristol inquiry, received enthusiastic backing from the New Labour government. Promoting patient empowerment in defiance of medical paternalism was central to Mr Blair's modernising agenda in the health service.

As Chief Medical Officer, Professor Donaldson was an active promoter of this agenda. Indeed, on the publication of the Alder Hey report in February 2001, Professor Donaldson appeared at a joint press conference with representatives of parents' organisations to indicate the medical establishment's commitment to challenging paternalism. In September 2001, Professor Donaldson approved a report (produced by a taskforce of which he was chair) promoting the notion of 'expert patients' – people suffering from chronic conditions whose long experience meant that they understood their diseases better than their doctors. Although this report insisted that the expert patients programme was 'not an anti-professional initiative', it took its place in a series of explicitly anti-professional initiatives (DH 2001). In December 2001, Professor Donaldson endorsed a report on ME/CFS produced by a committee dominated by representatives of patients' groups after most of the clinicians on the committee had resigned (DH 2002a, Fitzpatrick 2002). Professor Donaldson emphasised that the particular approach to the problems of chronic fatigue favoured by patients would be foisted on the medical profession. The elevation of subjective experience and consumer choice over medical science and expertise in these instances suited the government's purpose of introducing new mechanisms of professional regulation. But the government's populist strategy came to grief over MMR.

The problem that emerged with MMR is that individual choice cannot be reconciled with a mass childhood immunisation programme. Mass immunisation is a policy for preventing diseases at a population level. It requires that individual children be immunised, but decisions about what diseases to immunise against, when and how, can only be taken from the perspective of society as a whole, taking into account the nature of the diseases, the efficacy and availability of vaccines, and other factors. For every individual, the question of whether or not to be immunised depends on a judgement of the balance of benefits and risks. In the past, this was fairly straightforward: the risk of infectious disease was significant and the consequences of infection serious; the small risk of vaccine complications was widely regarded as one worth taking. The problem with MMR is that as the diseases it prevents have become uncommon, the risk of adverse effects, however rare, looms ever larger. However, once a significant proportion of the population opts out of immunisation, then the risk of the old diseases returning inevitably increases. The further, peculiar, problem of the recent MMR crisis is the emergence of a section of society prepared to opt out of immunisation (and accept the risk of disease for their children) in response to a risk that is entirely speculative.

The government's consistent promotion of an individualistic outlook meant that any appeal to a collective commitment to sustain 'herd immunity' was doomed. To criticise parents for making decisions that were selfish or self-seeking in the climate of consumer sovereignty promoted by New Labour seemed simply perverse. In the early 1990s Rogers and Pilgrim had noted that 'herd immunity carried little weight with parents committed to homeopathy' (Rogers, Pilgrim 1994: 47). Ten years later it carried little weight with anybody.

To justify its refusal to provide separate vaccines, the government was obliged to fall back on the arguments that its MMR policy was supported by expert medical advice and that there was no scientific evidence to justify the proposed alternative. This was true, but given its own tendency to disparage both the medical profession and scientific evidence it was not surprising that this approach made little impact on an increasingly cynical public. The demand for the right to choose separate vaccines had a ready appeal to a public whose right to choose schools and hospitals, methods of childbirth and dates for surgery, had been elevated into a principle of public policy. It was readily promoted by a range of private doctors and entrepreneurs who eagerly met the demand for separate vaccines resulting from the MMR scare. Profiting handsomely from the anti-MMR campaign, the proprietors of these clinics emerged as some of the most ardent supporters of Dr Wakefield's crusade.

While some parents demanded the right to expose their own children – and the children of others – to an increased risk of infectious diseases, some doctors (and some parents) began to look to the law to uphold children's rights to the protection provided by immunisation.

## Immunisation and the law

A requirement to produce evidence of immunisation at school entry, as in the USA, was suggested in the National Immunisation Study shortly after the introduction of MMR, but this was not introduced in Britain (Peckham et al 1989). The continuing decline in the uptake of MMR – and increasing concerns at the danger of outbreaks of measles – has revived discussion of various ways of making immunisation compulsory. For example, a resolution proposing compulsory vaccination was discussed at the annual conference of the British Medical Association in summer 2002 (where it was rejected). As some commentators have recommended the American system, it is worth briefly looking at what appears to be a distinctly authoritarian system, apparently at odds with US libertarian traditions.

Compulsory vaccination against smallpox was introduced in the USA (as in Britain) in the nineteenth century, and it was upheld against challenges in the Supreme Court in 1905 and 1922. Once the threat of smallpox receded, immunisation against other diseases proceeded on the basis of consent rather than coercion. However, in the 1970s a number of large-scale epidemics of measles, mainly affecting school-age children, led to efforts to enforce long-neglected statutes requiring vaccination as a condition for school entry (Orenstein, Hinman 1999). These pressures came, in part, from doctors and public health officials but also from parents of children who had been vaccinated, who recognised the risk resulting from the substantial numbers of 'free-riders' (who benefited from the herd immunity provided by those who were vaccinated, without themselves taking the risks, however small, of immunisation).

An outbreak of measles in Los Angeles in January 1977 proved a turning point. By March there were two deaths, three cases of encephalitis and many more of pneumonia. The public health authorities gave parents four weeks to get their children vaccinated or face exclusion from school. Within days of the target date, uptake was virtually 100 per cent. The authorities concluded that if this could be achieved in such a diverse and fragmented community, it could be achieved anywhere: 'The Los Angeles experience set the precedent that school exclusions and strict enforcement of immunisation requirements were possible and acceptable by most of the community' (Orenstein, Hinman 1999: S22). In the late 1970s and early 1980s, the extension and enforcement of school entry requirements in all the states of the union (there is still no federal legislation) resulted in a shift from chaotic responses to local epidemics to a comprehensive prevention policy. However, most states allow exemptions on religious grounds and some also allow 'philosophical' objections. Although, until recently, the numbers claiming such exemptions were negligible, there are signs that anti-immunisation sentiments are winning increasing support, particularly in prosperous areas (Feudtner, Marcuse 2001, McNeil 2002).

In their account of the role of school immunisation laws in the USA, Orenstein and Hinman emphasise that Americans accept this incursion on their cherished libertarian principles because of the high level of acceptance, by parents and doctors, of the rationale for mass childhood immunisation. The authors quote opinion polls indicating that hostility to the free-rider is as strong as approval for immunisation – and both far outweigh the notion that 'immunisation laws go against freedom of choice'. As Orenstein and Hinman put it, 'despite our citizens' love of freedom, mandatory immunisation is generally well accepted' (Orenstein, Hinman 1999: S19).

Although the American system has proved effective in ensuring the immunisation of school-age children, one consequence of the school-entry requirement is that many parents do not get their children immunised until shortly before they start school. This means that there is a substantial pool of children who are vulnerable to infection in the pre-school years, and this has resulted in persistent outbreaks of measles. By contrast, the consensual system in Britain has – at least until recently – been effective in ensuring that babies are protected from the early months of life, when the risks of infectious disease are often greater.

## Marital strife over MMR

In summer 2003 in Britain, a legal judgment that two girls should be given MMR and other vaccinations against the wishes of their mothers was welcomed by those who support a wider role for the law in enforcing public health policies, as in the USA. In the two separate cases, girls aged 4 and 10 lived with their mothers who had refused to have them vaccinated because of fears of adverse effects. Their fathers, who had parental responsibility and contact with the children although they were estranged from their children's mothers, applied to the court to enforce immunisation. Mr Justice Sumner described the medical evidence in favour of immunisation (given by paediatricians Dr Steven Conway and Professor Simon Kroll) as 'clear and persuasive' (Sumner 2003)

The judge was sharply critical of the expert evidence offered against immunisation by Dr Jayne Donegan, a GP and homeopath, whom he said had 'allowed her deeply held feelings on the subject of immunisation to overrule the duty she owes to the court'. He fully endorsed Dr Conway's comprehensive critique of her submission (which was based on references to 120 papers). She was accused of 'being confused in her thinking, lacking logic, minimising the duration of a disease, making statements lacking valid facts, ignoring the facts, ignoring the conclusion of papers, making implications without any scientific validation, giving a superficial impression of a paper, not presenting the counter-argument, quoting selectively from papers, and of providing in one instance no data and no facts to support her claim'. Sumner indicated that he was satisfied that Dr Conway 'was not over-critical' and he also upheld further criticisms by Professor Kroll concerning 'selective quotations' and 'unsubstantiated claims'. It was Dr Donegan's evidence that Lord Justice Sedley dismissed as 'junk science' at the subsequent appeal (Thorpe, Sedley, Evans 2003).

On the specific question of giving MMR as separate vaccines, Mr Justice Sumner concluded that he could see 'no advantage and much disadvantage' in this approach. In conclusion, 'while recognising the anxieties and feelings of the mothers', he 'was satisfied that age-appropriate immunisation was in both the children's best interests'. He thus ruled that both girls should receive the appropriate immunisations. While most commentators, both medical and legal, took the view that, on the basis of the evidence provided, the court had little alternative but to rule in favour of immunisation, most doctors would prefer to resolve conflicts of this sort by persuading parents of the benefits of vaccines and keeping the law out of the baby clinic.

Although the question of compulsion continues to arise in relation to MMR, on every occasion it has been seriously considered in recent years it has been dismissed. Thus the expert group on MMR convened by the Scottish Executive in 2001 concluded that it was 'not self-evident that it [compulsion] would lead to higher levels of immunisation' and opted to uphold the 'core principle that vaccines should be administered on a voluntary basis' (Scottish Executive 2002). In March 2003, the Department of Health indicated that it had no plans to alter its long-standing policy in favour of voluntary immunisation. In its guidebook on child-hood immunisation published in June 2003, the British Medical Association endorsed the principle that 'education not compulsion' was the key to high immunisation coverage (BMA 2003: 16).

## Government on the defensive

Parents' testimonies of their conviction that MMR had rendered their children autistic had great emotional force, especially when reinforced on television with selections from family videos showing the regression of thriving infants into disturbed autistic behaviour. The appearance in the media of these parents posed a difficult problem for doctors, scientists or politicians charged with upholding official immunisation policy: however persuasive their rational arguments in favour of MMR, they were no match for the images of anguished parents and their damaged children. Dr Wakefield's success in presenting himself as champion of families affected by autism gave him a crucial propaganda advantage over the immunisation authorities. While there was some criticism of prominent medical figures and Department of Health officials for appearing dismissive of Dr Wakefield's claims and intransigent in the face of the demand for separate vaccines, many doctors recognised that there was no alternative but to take a firm stand to uphold the integrity of the immunisation programme. Any concession to the anti-MMR campaign could have dealt a terminal blow to public confidence in the vaccine.

Dr Wakefield had another advantage. Although the medical consensus against his MMR–autism thesis was strong, there was a lack of conviction about publicly repudiating his position. The equivocation of Dr Wakefield's co-authors of the *Lancet* paper was one indication of this problem. Although some of the team declared support for MMR (Dr Wakefield was the only one of the *Lancet* paper's 13 signatories to support openly the call for separate vaccines), the gastroenterologists at the Royal Free Hospital (Professor John Walker-Smith, Drs Simon Murch and Mike Thomson) were keen to rescue the identification of 'autistic enterocolitis' (claimed to be a distinctive form of inflammatory bowel disease among autistic children) from the furore over MMR. But the reluctance of these experienced clinicians to distance themselves more sharply from Dr Wakefield provided a degree of cover for his anti-MMR crusade. At the Royal Free, it was left to Professor Brent Taylor, a community paediatrician not involved in the gastroenterology department, to make the case against Dr Wakefield. At the same time, given the intensity of the commitment of some parents of autistic children to the anti-MMR campaign, leading authorities in the world of autism were reluctant to appear unsympathetic to the Wakefield thesis. Those who did make public criticisms of Dr Wakefield's claims – notably Dr Eric Fombonne and Professor Christopher Gillberg – became, like Professor Taylor, targets of personal abuse by anti-MMR campaigners.

Equivocation among gastroenterologists and autism specialists left the initiative with Dr Wakefield, creating a problem for the immunisation authorities. They wanted to rebut Dr Wakefield's claims, but did not want to be seen to be victimising a hospital doctor with a growing media profile, and thus provide even more publicity for the anti-MMR campaign. The Department of Health's first response to the *Lancet* paper was to attempt to reassure the public that the MMR immunisation was safe. (Although the Department had several months' notice of the publication of Dr Wakefield's study, GPs and other frontline health workers still had to wait four weeks for the official response.) In 2001, as the demand for separate vaccines took off and Dr Wakefield raised further questions about the safety of MMR, the Department of Health launched a £3.5 million publicity campaign to bolster public confidence in MMR. But, by the early 1990s, official information about immunisation was already regarded with suspicion if not outright hostility by a significant section of the population. After the Operation Safeguard controversy (1994–95) and the 'mad cow' crisis (1996–98) there was a clear danger that any campaign of reassurance would be not merely ineffective, but counter-productive. The subsequent decline in uptake of MMR confirmed this fear. (It was therefore a considerable relief to frontline health workers that the Department of Health abandoned plans for a further publicity campaign in 2002 in favour of discreet local initiatives to bolster professional confidence in MMR.)

In despair at the steadily growing influence of the anti-MMR campaign, some medical commentators have come around to the view that it is only when epidemics of measles return that parents will appreciate the value of immunisation. 'Forget the carrot and bring out the stick', wrote teledoc Dr Mark Porter, 'what we need is an epidemic' (Porter 2003). From this perspective, any increase in notifications of measles is greeted as heralding an outbreak that may be used to encourage parents to get their children immunised. There is some suspicion that the 'outbreaks' in South London and the North East in early 2002 were little more than the small number of cases that still occur sporadically every year. However, given the concerns about the declining uptake of MMR, especially in London, these 'outbreaks' offered public health authorities an opportunity to promote fears about measles in the hope that these might overcome fears about autism and shift parents back towards MMR. Not surprisingly, this strategy appears to have been unsuccessful. Anxiety is not conducive to rational decision making: parents in the grip of contending fears are more likely to put off the decision, perhaps temporarily, perhaps indefinitely. Irrespective of measles outbreaks, MMR uptake in inner London has continued to decline.

In November 2002 concerns about the safety of Pavivac – a mumps vaccine imported from the Czech Republic by clinics giving separate vaccines – provided the government with another opportunity for a counter-scare. Sending an urgent message through the 'public health cascade' to all GPs and frontline health service workers, Dr Pat Troop, the Deputy Chief Medical Officer, announced the government's decision to suspend the import of Pavivac because of concerns over the 'manufacture, testing and storage' of the vaccine. In a lengthy 'Q&A' supplement to the urgent fax message, Dr Troop turned the prejudices of the anti-MMR campaign against the single mumps vaccine, raising the spectre of 'mad cow disease', the lack of safety data and even pointing out that the vaccine contained proteins derived from dogs. 'How come I wasn't advised about the presence of dog protein in Pavivac?' is one question Dr Troop suggested to the sort of parents who are not reluctant to assert their rights as consumers to full product information. She offered the answer that 'the doctor giving the vaccine is responsible for talking you through these issues'. On behalf of all those doctors who had spent hours talking anxious parents through the issues of MMR, Dr Troop was determined to make sure that the private clinic doctors selling separate vaccines for cash were now called to account.

In my view, this was all good fun and the anti-MMR campaigners richly deserved this dose of their own medicine. The squeals of outrage from Direct Health 2000 – one of the private clinics that has profited from the MMR scare – confirmed that the Department of Health's barbs had hit their target. Having been the beneficiaries of all the scaremongering over MMR, Direct Health 2000 was aggrieved to find itself at the receiving end of what it called 'appalling scaremongering' over the mumps vaccine. In July 2003 the Department of Health closed down two private clinics (in Elstree and Sheffield) when they were discovered to be in violation of basic standards and referred their clinical director to the General Medical Council. Although this action was widely welcomed by doctors in public health and primary care, the response of parents who had taken their children to these clinics was one of continuing resentment at the government for not making these vaccines available on the NHS.

The real casualties of this war of scares were parents whose children were due for vaccination. Competing fears may have made them more anxious – and more angry – but they did not encourage them to have their children vaccinated with the MMR.

# 4

# AGE OF ANXIETY

There are many insults to the human body as a result of life
in the last decade of the twentieth century. Pesticides, agri-
cultural chemicals, antibiotics, preservatives, pollution or
junk food *may* be responsible for the changing pattern of
this serious and distressing childhood condition [autism].
(Richard Barr and Kirsten Limb, solicitors leading parents'
litigation against MMR; Limb, Barr 1998: 31)

For most parents, our children are everything to us: our
hopes, our ambitions, our future. Our children are cherished
and loved.
(Tony Blair, Foreword, *Every Child Matters*, Green Paper,
September 2003; www.dfes.gov.uk/everychildmatters/)

The MMR–autism scare emerged in Britain in the late 1990s at a
time of unprecedented social anxiety over environmental threats to
health and safety. The perception that antibiotics and pesticides – as
well as immunisations – may be to blame for the apparent rise in the
prevalence of autism may sound preposterous. Indeed, it is preposterous: not only is there no evidence for this proposition, it is made
in relation to three products of modern science and technology that
have each made a major contribution to improving and prolonging
human life over the past century. Yet these have been casually listed,
together with 'pollution', as 'insults' to the human body, in a document published by a prestigious firm of London solicitors. Although
we may be horrified to read such absurdities in what purports to be
an 'information pack' for parents, we can no longer be shocked,
because such statements have become commonplace. The addition
of 'junk food' to the litany of environmental 'insults' indicates the
range of threats against which modern consumers must protect
themselves and their children.

Whereas early environmental campaigners expressed concern about the impact of human intervention on nature, contemporary anxieties focus on perceived environmental threats to humanity. The fact that even beneficial products of modern society, such as antibiotics and vaccines, are now regarded as potential causes of serious diseases reflects the degree of alienation experienced by many and the feelings of vulnerability that result. Although by objective criteria people in Western societies today live longer and healthier lives than at any time in human history, we are uniquely preoccupied by our health and the measures considered necessary to preserve it. Anxieties about health are expressed in the fashion for physical exercise (devoted to fitness rather than to fun), the popularity of health screening programmes, diets and supplements. Yet these, and numerous other health-related activities, do not appear to alleviate existential anxieties. The resonance for an apparently endless series of health scares over issues from mobile phone masts to GM foods reflects the high level of free-floating anxiety in society.

Parents' anxieties are often projected onto their children. In his foreword to the government's Green Paper on children, Tony Blair articulates the contemporary worship of children in a characteristically sentimental form (see page 39). But, as the MMR controversy confirms, children have become a focus of fears as well as of hopes. It also reveals that in the current climate of health-related anxieties some parents are prepared to forgo immunisation for their children and expose them to a real risk of infectious diseases in response to a speculative risk of autism.

Tony Blair has hailed the establishment of NHS Direct – a 24-hour, nurse-led, telephone advice service – as one of the major achievements of his first thousand days as Prime Minister (*Guardian*, 26 February 2000). This symbolic 'one-to-one' communication between the anxious citizen worried about a health-related problem and a proxy for the caring, listening Prime Minister, is a potent image of the new therapeutic relationship between the government and the people. The success of NHS Direct reveals both the need of the vulnerable individual for solace and reassurance, and the need of a government that lacks authority and legitimacy to establish points of contact with an increasingly atomised and alienated electorate. However, although a call to NHS Direct may suffice to quell individual anxieties, government reassurances over MMR have failed to persuade a substantial body of parents that it is safe.

While the 'mad cow disease' scandal is commonly blamed for undermining trust in government and in science, this perception of the BSE/CJD issue is more a result of a new climate of suspicion and cynicism than a reason for it. First, let us look more closely at some of the social and political factors that have contributed to the feelings of insecurity and vulnerability that have found expression in relation to immunisation and other health issues in recent years.

## The children of Thatcherism

The transformation of the political landscape in Britain over the past 20 years reflects a wider process of fragmentation. When I was a medical student in the 1970s, it was customary to open the presentation of a case history on a ward round by indicating the patient's age, sex and occupation; occupation, even if retired, was a cipher for social class, which was really all the consultant needed to know. But this was in the days before chronic mass unemployment, flexible labour markets and flexible identities. A couple of years ago I found myself at a lunchtime meeting at the local hospital at which the case of a patient of mine was being presented to illustrate an unusual condition of some academic interest. I was surprised to find that she was introduced as 'a 48-year-old Rastafarian'. When I saw her next in the surgery, I said, 'I never knew you were a Rasta'. 'No, man', came the reply, 'I just had my hair in locks and they put that down on the form'. New forms of identity, in terms of ethnicity, sexuality or lifestyle may sound more exotic, but they tend to be less stable and cohesive than the ones they have replaced (Malik 1996: 247–52).

While the living standards of people on benefits may have stagnated, those of anybody with any sort of earned income have tended to improve. However, higher pay may have been achieved at the cost of declining job security and workplace control and as trades unions and other protections have been weakened. One consequence of the changing character of relations in the workplace is the epidemic of work stress (Wainwright, Calnan 2002). In the course of successive booms and recessions, insecurity has spread to every level of the labour market, to the public sector as well as the private sector. Today nobody has a job for life; and nobody can rely on a secure pension, any more than they can be confident about getting a decent education for their children in state schools or prompt and efficient medical treatment through the NHS (Toynbee, Walker 2001).

In the early 1970s our lectures were disrupted by the power cuts of the three-day week, and strikes and demonstrations were commonplace. There may have been a high level of conflict between trades unions and employers, but these were also rival cultures of solidarity, providing collective strength as well as collective bargaining. This world came to an end in the course of the 1980s as the labour movement and the Left collapsed and the establishment lost the enemies against which it had united its forces over two centuries. The resulting loss of cohesion and morale was reflected in the rapid decline in status of a range of key British institutions. As well as the Conservative Party, the Monarchy, the Church of England, the House of Lords, even the BBC and the Civil Service have been riven by internal strife as their public esteem has plummeted. Meanwhile, the level of popular disengagement from the political process was expressed in the 59 per cent turn-out in the 2001 general election – the lowest since the Second World War (Butler, Kavanagh 2001).

The combined effect of these social and political changes was to produce a society of increasingly atomised individuals. By crushing socialism and rolling back the state, Margaret Thatcher destroyed traditional collective organisations. But instead of creating a climate of opinion that celebrated individual responsibility and autonomy, what emerged was a culture of complaint and victimhood, which elevated the values of safety over those of risk taking. This culture was responsive to health scares of any sort; it was particularly vulnerable to scares that affected children.

The impact of these scares was heavily influenced by the new modes of family life that emerged in the late twentieth century. Falling rates of marriage and rising rates of divorce have reduced the stability of the family in modern Britain. The statistics of family breakdown are familiar (National Statistics 2003: 41–52). The proportion of men who are married declined from 71 per cent in 1971 to 54 per cent in 2001; for women the rates declined from 65 per cent to 52 per cent. Over the same period the proportion of the population who were divorced increased by a factor of eight for men and nine for women. In 1971 a quarter of men and a fifth of women were single; this rose to a third of men and a quarter of women by 2000. One of the most dramatic trends in recent decades has been the growth in people living alone: single-person households more than doubled from 3 million in 1971 to 6.2 million in 2001; 29 per cent of households now contain only one person (National Statistics 2003: 42–3).

As families have become smaller and less stable, children have become both increasingly precious and more problematic. While Britain's relatively high rate of teenage pregnancy is a target of a high-profile government agency and a frequent subject of public discussion, a perhaps more significant social trend is that towards later childbearing. The average age of mothers at childbirth has increased by three years since 1971 and is now over age 29. The average age of women at the birth of their first child is now over 27, while first-time fathers are now, on average, over 30 (National Statistics 2003: 51). Meanwhile average family size has steadily declined: the stereotypical figure of 2.4 children is now closer to 1.5.

For older parents with only one or two children, the process of having and rearing children also tends to be taken more seriously than in the past. Conceptions are more often planned; pregnancies demand attendance (often jointly) at antenatal clinics and classes; modes of birth are carefully chosen and deliveries routinely attended by fathers. Regarded as a middle class fad when I was a medical student, and guaranteed to produce an upward roll of the midwife's eyeballs, this has rapidly become universal (Mander 2004). Every stage of infant and childhood development is carefully – and often anxiously – observed and monitored. Many parents have substantial collections of magazines, pamphlets and books covering the whole range of health issues involved in having children. Even if parents only read the information officially provided to cover pregnancy, childbirth and early childcare, they would probably know more about these subjects than I did when I qualified as a doctor. And once they have survived infancy, there is the problem of getting them educated. . . .

Today's parents are also often preoccupied with child safety. Although this has produced a flourishing market in everything from household intercoms to 'baby on board' signs for cars to soft playground surfaces, it has also raised concerns about the dangers of overprotecting children. While today's parents are generally able to lavish material resources on their children (to a degree that often appals their grandparents), providing them with time may be a bigger problem. The resulting difficulties, especially for middle-class mothers, of 'having it all', have been expressed in numerous novels, magazine articles, newspaper features and television programmes, as well as in academic studies (Nicolson 2002).

Traditionally regarded as a haven from the pressures of the world of work, the modern family has become the focus of intense public anxiety and increasingly the target of professional intervention. Far from being regarded in a benign light, there has been a tendency more recently to regard the family as a cloistered world of domestic violence, where the physical and sexual abuse of children is commonplace. While the abduction of children by a stranger remains a potent fear, it has been eclipsed by the terror of abuse by somebody much closer to home, if not in the home. Despite the proliferation of police checks on childcare workers of any sort, parents are now reluctant to trust anybody with their children, sometimes even themselves. While the government seeks to promote parenting classes for wayward teenagers, they are most popular with older, middle-class parents who feel the need for professional tuition in matters of childrearing.

A way of illustrating the changing climate of opinion around issues of health and safety in Britain between the 1970s and 1990s is to contrast the public responses to two major scandals: thalidomide and 'mad cow disease'. The drug thalidomide was withdrawn from the market in 1961 after a number of babies, whose mothers had taken the drug as a sedative in early pregnancy, were born with absent limbs and other serious abnormalities. A scandal erupted in the 1970s over the drug companies' attempts to avoid paying appropriate compensation to the victims' families. Although Bovine Spongiform Encephalopathy (BSE) was first identified in cattle in 1988, it was not until 1996 that it was recognised that this condition was transmissible to humans in the form of 'variant' Creuzefeldt-Jakob Disease (CJD), a rapidly fatal brain disorder. The ensuing scandal concerned the issue of whether adequate steps were taken by those in authority to safeguard the public or to warn of the dangers of this terrible disease.

## Thalidomide: a real medical scandal

Developed by the German company Grunenthal, thalidomide was first marketed in Germany in 1957 and rapidly exported around the world. In Britain it was licensed to the Distillers company, which launched it in 1958.

In 1961, doctors in Australia, Germany and Britain independently noted an alarming increase in babies being born with hitherto very rare combinations of abnormalities of the limbs, eyes and ears, sometimes together with defects of the gastro-intestinal and genito-urinary systems. This pattern was first linked to thalidomide by William McBride, an Australian obstetrician, and when this link was also suspected in Germany, the drug was withdrawn. By this time, thalidomide had been sold in 46 countries: an estimated 10,000 children were born with some resulting abnormality, more than 500 in Britain. Because of what was widely regarded as the bureaucratic and conservative character of the US regulatory authorities (the Food and Drugs Administration), thalidomide was never licensed in the USA (although a few cases of fetal abnormalities resulted from large-scale, but poorly regulated trials)[1].

The thalidomide scandal erupted over the issue of compensation. In 1972 it emerged that the drug companies were secretly persuading families to accept modest sums in out-of-court settlements in return for abandoning further action. Furthermore, they invoked the principles of commercial secrecy to prevent investigation of their pre-marketing safety studies and secured court injunctions against attempts by newspapers – notably the *Sunday Times* – to expose their activities. In 1973, a parents' campaign, supported by sympathetic politicians and investigative journalists, provoked a revolt by Distillers' shareholders (including local councils and insurance companies), which finally forced the company to make a satisfactory financial settlement. Because of continuing legal disputes, it was some years before the full story about thalidomide could be told. Yet when it finally emerged, few would dispute the judgement of the *Sunday Times* Insight Team that it was one of 'greed and indifference, of incompetence and evasion' (*Sunday Times* Insight Team 1979: cover).

Thalidomide was promoted by Grunenthal and Distillers as a superior drug to existing tranquillisers: the manufacturers claimed that 'it was non-toxic, had no side-effects, and was completely safe for pregnant women'. Unfortunately 'none of these statements, announced by the drug companies and accepted by the doctors, was true' (*Sunday Times* Insight Team 1979: 10). Nor was it true, as the companies claimed, that it was not customary at the time to test such drugs on pregnant animals: it was just that the companies concerned had failed to conduct adequate toxicity tests. The companies tried to intimidate doctors who blew the whistle on thalidomide, and worked assiduously to avoid taking responsibility for the debacle. In this they were assisted in Britain by the government, the medical establishment, the judiciary and much of the press. Legal constraints prevented investigation of drug company files and also prevented the press from reporting on the matter. 'Secrecy cast a long shadow in the thalidomide affair', commented the Insight Team, 'first over the discovery over what went wrong, medically and legally, and then over the publication of the truth' (*Sunday Times* Insight Team 1979: 13). The thalidomide story was 'a story about a cover-up as well as about a drug disaster'.

---

1  The following is largely derived from the *Sunday Times* Insight Team's book (1979), supplemented by the later accounts of Stephens and Brynner (2001) and Shah (2001).

Although the conclusion of the Insight Team in 1979 was that 'it could happen again', a number of consequences resulting from the scandal appeared to make such a disaster less likely (*Sunday Times* Insight Team 1979: 314). Perhaps most importantly, it made pregnant women more reluctant to take any medication and doctors less enthusiastic to prescribe it. The thalidomide affair also vindicated the FDA's tough regulatory stance, which was further reinforced in the USA and more closely emulated in Britain and elsewhere (Shah 2001). It encouraged the reform of personal injury litigation in favour of victims of corporate negligence, the subject of a subsequent Royal Commission in Britain. Although there was no formal change in the legal status of the press, the moral victory of the *Sunday Times* in the thalidomide case undoubtedly advanced the cause of press freedom against claims of commercial secrecy or contempt.

Looking back on the thalidomide scandal more than two decades later, it is also worth noting consequences that did *not* ensue. Despite the exposure of venality, deception, intimidation and corruption in the pharmaceutical industry (with catastrophic consequences for thousands of families) and the complicity of much of the medical, legal and political establishment (which might have deprived the victims of due compensation), there was no breakdown in public confidence in any of these agencies or institutions. No doubt the scandal seriously damaged the reputations of the companies and the key figures involved. Yet public confidence in general in scientists and doctors, in capitalist enterprise and government regulation, in the press and the judiciary, remained high. It survived the revelation of serious inadequacies in all parties involved in what was widely regarded as an exceptional case.

(A fascinating footnote to the thalidomide story has a bearing on the MMR controversy [Rodier 2000]. Around 5 per cent of the children affected by thalidomide were found to be autistic – a rate about 30 times higher than that in the general population. Furthermore, most of these children were born with abnormalities of the external ears, but not of the arms or legs, indicating that the damage to the developing fetus had occurred very early in gestation – between 20 and 24 days – before many women even know they are pregnant. This suggests that whatever other environmental agents may contribute to the emergence of autism, they are likely to act at this very early stage of fetal development, rather than, as suggested by the MMR theory, in early childhood.)

## The real 'mad cow' scandal: nobody lied

The emergence of BSE was not caused by a drug, but was, most probably, the result of intensive farming practices, notably the use of 'meat and bone meal' feeds for cattle. Although the mechanism through which the infectious agent, or 'prion', that causes BSE is transmitted to humans, where it produces variant CJD, remains obscure, there is now little doubt that these diseases are caused by the same organism. Mercifully, vCJD remains rare: between its recognition in 1995 and the end of 2003, there had been 146 cases and 139 deaths in the UK; as the number of new cases has settled to less than 20 each year, early projections of a major epidemic have been abandoned (www.cjd.ed.ac.uk/figures.htm).

The contrast with the thalidomide scandal is immediately apparent: a much smaller scale of human injury caused a much greater economic, social and political impact. The fall in demand for British beef and the restriction of British exports had a devastating impact on beef farming and the associated food processing industry. The panic about beef – and continuing alarms about beef products used to prepare vaccines, beef on the bone, contaminated blood transfusions, surgical instruments – ensured a continuing level of anxiety over the next few years. Popular animosity over the Conservative Government's handling of the 'mad cow' crisis contributed to the New Labour landslide victory at the 1997 general election. A consensus rapidly emerged that the BSE/CJD affair had precipitated a major loss of public confidence in scientists, doctors, civil servants and politicians.

However, if we look back over the period following the emergence of BSE, there is scant evidence that wrongdoing by any of the professionals involved contributed significantly to the epidemic of vCJD (Fitzpatrick 1998). In 1988, the government appointed an inquiry into BSE under the Oxford zoologist Professor Richard Southwood. The leading scientific experts on this committee took the view that the transmission of BSE to humans was highly improbable. All previous experience with diseases of this sort (transmissible spongiform encephalopathies) indicated that there was a strong 'species barrier' preventing such spread: 'scrapie', for example, had been endemic among sheep in Britain for hundreds of years, but had never spread to man. Yet the committee explicitly recognised that if such transmission were to occur the consequences could be catastrophic. Hence it recommended a series of precautionary measures to prevent this – measures that were implemented before the inquiry report was published. These included a ban on 'meat and bone meal' from the human food chain and arrangements to destroy carcasses of cattle with BSE. A ban on 'specified bovine offals' – tissues such as brain, spinal cord, spleen, tonsils and thymus, which were known to contain potentially infective prions – followed in 1989. The Southwood Inquiry also proposed a high-level 'spongiform encephalopathy advisory committee' to advise government and the establishment of a surveillance unit to look out for any signs of transmission to humans (Southwood 1989).

In response to occasional suggestions in the late 1980s and early 1990s that BSE might become a threat to humans, politicians and civil servants echoed the scientific consensus expressed in the Southwood report and insisted that 'beef is safe'. The most dramatic public display of this conviction took place in May 1990 when then Agriculture Minister John Selwyn Gummer tried to force his infant daughter Cordelia to eat a hamburger to show his confidence in British beef. (The impact was somewhat spoiled when she refused to eat it.) In retrospect, politicians and civil servants were criticised for playing down health risks out of a desire to avoid a health scare and the resulting damage to farming and the food supply industries. But, given the scientific consensus that the danger to humans was remote, the inclination to reassure the public, and to safeguard trade and jobs, was entirely understandable and reasonable. With the benefit of hindsight from a more risk-averse age, they might have modified their reassurances that 'beef is safe' by saying that 'there is at present no evidence to suggest that beef is unsafe', but this would have done nothing to deter the spread of the disease.

In early 1996 the CJD surveillance unit, based in Edinburgh, identified the first cases of vCJD. The appearance of ten cases of a new, rapidly progressive form of CJD that seemed to particularly affect young people was a shock to the scientists. A nightmare scenario, of the sort that is always being predicted by some prophet of doom and always being dismissed by serious scientists, was unfolding before their eyes. The horror of the scientists was transmitted via the spongiform encephalopathy advisory committee to the heart of government, where it led directly to the notorious 20 March 1996 joint statement to the House of Commons by Health Secretary Stephen Dorrell and Agriculture Minister Douglas Hogg. For the first time the government admitted that 'the most likely explanation' for these cases of CJD was 'exposure to BSE'. Apart from drawing public attention to the BSE–CJD link, in a way that precipitated a major public panic and the collapse of the British beef trade, neither the parliamentary statement nor that subsequently issued by Chief Medical Officer Kenneth Calman, had any public health value. The only specific measures introduced were a minor tightening-up of the procedures introduced in 1988 and 1989.

After New Labour came to power in 1997, a major inquiry was established under Lord Justice Phillips into the BSE/CJD affair. This reported, at voluminous length, in October 2000 (Phillips Report 2000). After an exhaustive review of all aspects of the affair, the report criticised a number of senior scientists, doctors and civil servants and blamed the failure to act rapidly in response to events on a combination of complacency, secrecy and Whitehall infighting.

It is important to put these failings in context. The key events in the BSE/CJD story were the emergence of a new disease in cattle and its transmission to humans: both were more freak biological accidents than the results of human perfidy. In the course of human history and its close association with the domestication of animals a number of diseases have crossed over, causing measles, smallpox, influenza (McNeil 1976: 54). The distinctive feature of the 'mad cow' epidemic was how rapidly it was identified and measures taken to deal with it. Whatever mistakes were made after 1988/89 are unlikely to have had any effect on the number of cases of vCJD: in all probability, these resulted from transmission from infected beef in the mid-1980s, before measures were taken to curtail the BSE epidemic and to safeguard the human food chain.

The assertion that 'the government lied to us' over BSE/CJD has become a standard rebuttal to official reassurances about any subject, including MMR. Yet, even according to the Phillips Report, which was not reluctant to chastise officials for being secretive and bureaucratic, there was no evidence of deliberate deception. (In contrast with thalidomide, investigative journalism played no part in the BSE/CJD affair.) What happened over BSE/CJD was that a freak biological event – an unfortunate accident – led to the emergence and transmission of a new disease. Even if scientists and officials had been more open and efficient in acknowledging the resulting problems, this would have done nothing to prevent the spread of the disease among humans. Although there was nothing in the BSE/CJD affair to compare with the grave derelictions of responsibility by the private corporations and public institutions that were exposed over thalidomide, the public impact was far greater. In the 1990s, when popular confidence in science, medicine and government was already running low and anxieties over health issues were running high, the 'mad cow' crisis served to reinforce prevailing prejudices. Although nobody lied to anybody over 'mad cow disease', the popularity of the mantra that 'they lied to us' confirmed the level of popular disillusionment with official expertise in all forms.

## The immune system as metaphor

The concept of the 'immune system' is at the centre of contemporary concerns about immunisation, as it is of wider discussions about health. Indeed, as we shall see in Chapter 6, it is also believed by some to play an important role in autism. Patients often come into the surgery, saying 'Doctor, I think my immune system is suppressed'. They are unsure whether this may result from their busy lifestyle, their failure to follow a healthy diet, or whether they are the victims of some occult viral or yeast infection, allergy or some other malign influence. They wonder whether some combination of these factors explains their recurrent coughs and colds or their general feeling of tiredness and malaise. Others fear that their immune system has become 'overloaded' by unspecified environmental toxins or pollutants or as a result of antibiotics or immunisations. The spectre of HIV/AIDS – a mysterious but deadly virus that destroys immunity – has had a major influence on contemporary ideas of health and disease. As the American social anthropologist Emily Martin puts it, 'the immune system has moved to the very centre of our culture's conception of health' (Martin 1994: 186).

In her book, *Flexible Bodies: The role of immunity in American culture from the days of polio to the age of Aids*, Martin explores 'the emergence of the immune system as a field in terms of which all manner of questions about health are given meaning and measured' (Martin 1994: xvii). She gives a fascinating account of the spread of concepts of immunity, from popular scientific publications in the 1980s to the 'saturation' of the mainstream media in the 1990s. By then every member of the White House household was said to have an auto-immune disease (that is, George and Barbara Bush, and the dog), TV car ads featured claims that some model was an 'antibody for auto accidents', and immune dysfunction was invoked to explain virtually every disorder – of the body, the mind, and even of society.

Martin identifies a shift from the use of military metaphors, in which the immune system defends the self against enemy attack, to more holistic notions of the body as a 'complex regulatory system' within the larger world order (Martin 1994: 122). The sense that everything about your health is connected to everything that exists and that it is your responsibility to manage and control these interactions results in the paradox of 'empowered powerlessness': 'feeling responsible for everything and powerless at the same time' (Martin 1994: 122):

> Once we see the healthy body as if it were a complex system teetering along the path of life pretty well most of the time, but always on the verge of falling over the edge into catastrophe, a pervasive sense of anxiety that is difficult to assuage seems inevitable.
>
> (Martin 1994: 135)

Popular concepts of immunity reflect the prevailing sense of individual vulnerability in an age of anxiety.

The term 'immune system' is now so familiar that it has the aura of a medical or scientific concept that has been around since the seventeenth century. In fact, the term is scarcely 30 years old: it was first used by the immunologist Niels Jerne at a symposium in New York in 1967 (Moulin 1989: 293–4). As Anne Marie Moulin, an historian of immunology, explains, the term was introduced as a pragmatic device to hold together two contending factions within the discipline. On the one hand were those who held that specialised cells (lymphocytes) were the key factor in fighting off infection; on the other were those who emphasised the role of circulating antibodies (immunoglobulins). As Jerne put it, 'the immune system of an adult person can most simply be described as an ensemble of $10^{12}$ lymphocytes and $10^{10}$ antibody molecules' (Moulin 1989: 295).

'Why was the term immune system accepted so widely and so rapidly?' asks Moulin. She attributes its success to its capacity to convey different meanings, to its 'linguistic versatility'. Given that 'system' was traditionally understood as 'tissue', the term implied an anatomical basis for immunity (which was, in fact, very ill-defined). In modern usage, the concept 'system' implied structure and invited mathematical modelling. It also referred to a body of knowledge, rooted in the past and carrying great promise for the future, and conferred legitimacy on the emerging discipline of immunology. For Moulin, the immune system 'was a kind of metaphor' – one that 'solved the need of communication not only between cells, but between the professionals of immunity'. If, as Moulin notes, 'in the 1970s, the *immune system* provided a trendy title for numerous lectures, articles, books, reviews', in the 1990s, the term moved beyond the world of science and entered a new phase of popularity in the public realm.

The 'linguistic versatility' of the term 'immune system' was also the key to its crossover into vernacular notions of science. But the content of the concept also changed in the course of this transition. Although the term was borrowed from the science of immunology, its new meaning was filled out with ideas derived from influential contemporary trends, notably environmentalism, alternative health and New Age mysticism. At a time when these social movements expressed a profound pessimism about the prospects for the planet and a misanthropic outlook on humanity, the concept of an enfeebled immune system reflected the widespread sense of fragile individuality.

In a survey of popular literature on 'ME/CFIDS' (myalgic encephalomyelitis/chronic fatigue immune deficiency syndrome), psychiatrist Simon Wessely and colleagues note that the concept of the immune system plays a central role:

> 'Weakening' of the immune system is at the heart of the popular models of ME/CFIDS – this can be the result of viral infections, nutritional deficiencies, chemicals, candida, and so on – indeed, one of the ways in which the popular literature acknowledges a role for psychological factors and even depression, is via their alleged effect on the immune system.
>
> (Wessely et al 1998: 321)

The concept of a threatened immune system also provides a link with other 'unexplained somatic syndromes' – food allergies, multiple chemical sensitivity, irritable bowel syndrome, fibromyalgia. The authors draw attention to the way in which scientific concepts, such as the immune system, have become parodied in the popular literature, which reflects an overriding sense of disquiet about the state of the environment.

Advocacy groups formed in relation to disorders attributed to immune dysfunction have made extensive use of parodies of the scientific concept of immunity. In a book subtitled 'Environmental illness and the struggle over medical knowledge' two US professors of sociology describe the process of 'non-physicians constructing medical explanations for their physical symptoms and miseries' (Kroll-Smith, Hugh Floyd 1997). They welcome this as part of 'a wider, more inclusive trend', in which 'ordinary people borrow expert rhetorics, locating them in non-expert systems, and working to politicise what is routinely considered natural' (Kroll-Smith,

Hugh Floyd 1997: xiii). Although the authors consider this 'an alternative strategy for the construction of rational knowledge in late modern society', it may also be characterised as the selective use of scientific concepts to confer legitimacy on a political act – the claim for the status of illness or victimhood (with all its benefits and disadvantages) for a particular group in society. The authors also claim that 'lay expertise is emerging as an alternative form of rationality, one that begins and ends with concrete human, indeed physical, experiences' (Kroll-Smith, Hugh Floyd 1997: 7). But the only form of rationality that begins and ends with 'concrete experiences' is the crudest empiricism, which has never been of much value in the understanding and treatment of human disease.

Following trends in sociology and anthropology, it has become fashionable to reinterpret the thinking of primitive societies and lay wisdom in contemporary societies as distinctive forms of rationality, with their own claims to the status of science. However, as the embryologist Lewis Wolpert observes, traditional cosmologies are closed and uncritical, they acknowledge no alternatives and are incapable of confessing ignorance (Wolpert 1992: 35–55). Nor have they made any contribution to what we understand as science – the distinctive product of Classical Greece and the Enlightenment. Philosophers who ignore the achievements of modern science, remain agnostic about whether a particular theory is right or wrong and deny the concept of progress, miss the essence of the scientific enterprise. It is ironic that scientific ideas that have become to some degree popularised in contemporary societies, such as elements of quantum theory or concepts of immunity, tend to be interpreted in a mystical or magical way. As Wolpert argues, 'scientific modes of thought are psychologically uncomfortable, whereas magic may be seen as a means of defending the self against the hostile world which is not easily given up' (Wolpert 1992: 141).

'Auto-immunity', the idea that the human body generates a destructive immune response to its own tissues, is another concept that has a popular resonance (Clark 1995). Although the possibility of auto-immunity was first suggested by Paul Erhlich, one of the pioneers of immunology at the turn of the nineteenth to twentieth centuries, it was first confirmed in the 1940s and identified as the cause of a human disease (Hashimoto's thyroiditis) in 1956. Over the next twenty years a number of diseases – including insulin-dependent diabetes, haemolytic anaemia, myasthenia gravis, systemic lupus erythematosus – were found to have an auto-immune basis. Over the same period, numerous other disorders of unknown cause were attributed to auto-immunity: as one authority puts it, 'the medical literature of the 1960s and 1970s is filled with references to so-called autoimmune diseases' (Clark 1995: 122). In more recent years, as we shall consider further in Chapter 6, theories of auto-immunity have been invoked to explain autism, and the alleged adverse effects of various vaccinations. In these cases, the popular appeal of the notion of human self-destructiveness seems to be a more significant explanation for the influence of these theories than any scientific evidence adduced to support them.

Over the past decade parodies of the scientific concept of immunity, once the preserve of a bohemian fringe, have won widespread popularity. They are articulated and promoted by practitioners of diverse schools of alternative health, by promoters of austere lifestyles and esoteric diets, and by purveyors of vitamins, antioxidants, trace minerals, herbal and homeopathic remedies. They are no longer confined to specialist magazines, but now permeate the mainstream media. They are also increasingly expressed in scientific (or at least pseudo-scientific) jargon, giving anti-scientific prejudices the aura of scientific legitimacy.

High on the list of what many now regard as potential dangers to the immune system are antibiotics and immunisations. Both are regarded as damaging to the operation of natural processes of immunity and as potential causes of illness. As I have discovered in numerous discussions with patients who hold these beliefs, to inquire as to how antibiotics and immunisations might damage the immune system is to miss the point. These beliefs are not derived from a study of immunology as a science, but arise from a general feeling of vulnerability to a particular sort of danger. This no longer arises from nature as such (in the way that in the past people feared infectious diseases) but from the products of human intervention in nature (antibiotics, vaccines). The linguistic versatility of the concept of the immune system can no longer reconcile people speaking different languages.

The current controversy over MMR reveals the influence of the immune system as metaphor. Indeed it appears that elements of the popular parody of the scientific concept of the immune system were adopted by Dr Wakefield – at the outset, at least, a researcher within the medical mainstream. As a result, the challenge to medical orthodoxy has appeared to take the form of a division within medicine, rather than an attack from without. The confusions around the concept of the immune system contribute to what often appears like a dialogue of Babel in the MMR–autism debate.

## Facts are not enough

Our baby clinic is much older than the health centre. A pre-war photograph recently discovered in the council archives shows a 'Maternity and Child Welfare Centre' located in a converted terrace house on the site now occupied by the health centre (built in the early 1970s). Centres like this were first established around the time of the First World War in response to concerns about poor standards of nutrition and health among the nation's children. We now see 20 or more babies and toddlers at each clinic, for developmental checks, advice about feeding, sleeping and other problems, and for immunisations. The clinic reflects the diversity of the area. We have teenage mothers and mothers in their 40s; professional parents living in gentrified Victorian housing and unemployed parents from neglected council estates; we have traditional Hackney families, and families from many ethnic minority and immigrant groups, from (unevenly) assimilated Irish, Jewish and Caribbean people, to newly arriving Bangladeshis, Turks, Kurds and Polish Gypsies.

The baby clinic is a noisy but generally cheerful place. Whereas patients attending normal surgeries tend to be ill or in some form of distress, in the baby clinic the babies are usually well and their parents are happy to bring them along to a familiar place where they often meet neighbours and friends. However, in recent years, largely as a result of the MMR controversy, the baby clinic has lost some of its relaxed and harmonious atmosphere. Fears about the dangers of vaccines, promoted by the media, have made parents anxious, uncertain and confused. As the public debate has gathered momentum, households in which MMR is imminent have been drawn into the nationwide controversy. In our clinic we have noticed tensions between fathers and mothers (often, fathers, who in the past rarely attended baby clinics and probably knew little about what immunisations their child was receiving, now have strong opinions about MMR), between parents and the wider community of family and friends (who now probably include at least one fervent anti-MMR advocate). We have also noticed increasing tensions between parents and doctors, as parents take offence at what they perceive as professional pressure to conform to the immunisation programme. Some parents are resentful at the denial of the choice of separate vaccines and angry at attempts to make them feel guilty about refusing or postponing the triple vaccine. Although our rates of vaccine uptake have fallen, the amount of time taken up in discussions about immunisation is much greater.

One result is that the baby clinic invariably runs late: all staff are guaranteed a late lunch.

The strength of emotions underlying the rejection of MMR is confirmed by the difficulty we experience in persuading parents who have adopted this outlook to change their minds. This is why all the efforts of the Department of Health and leading medical and health promotion agencies to provide information and reassurance about MMR have proved largely ineffectual, if not counterproductive. Indeed, research in Australia suggests that when parents were presented with factual information about risks and benefits of immunisation, they tended to become more committed to their resistance (Meszaros et al 1996). In their discussion of parental responses to press coverage of immunisation issues in Australia, Julie-Anne Leask and colleagues noted that the appeal of anti-vaccination claims lay in their 'underlying reference' to 'a canopy of more general discourses' about 'cover-up and conspiracy, manipulation by venal private enterprise interests, governments with totalitarian agendas and the back-to-nature idyll' (Leask et al 1998, 2000).

It is clear that, for some parents, the decision to refuse MMR has little to do with MMR as such. Thus, it is not unusual to find that, while some parents who have decided against it are quite well informed about the case against immunisation, many are not. Their decision is not based on a study of the particularities of MMR, but the result of the wider set of attitudes noted by these Australian researchers – attitudes that became increasingly widespread in a section of the educated middle classes during the course of the 1990s. They were expressed in a growing suspicion and distrust of science and medicine, of capitalist corporations and mainstream politicians, and a general mood of anger and resentment. Middle-class discontents became apparent around a range of political issues: fuel prices, student loans, blood sports and the invasion of Iraq. Yet MMR provided a focus for protest that was both intensely personal and highly political. It brought together issues of health and child welfare that were both already central preoccupations of a highly individuated society.

The controversy over immunisation allowed scope for individual initiative, at least in the form of a gesture of defiance, which was generally lacking in the public sphere. If you could do nothing about the oppressive culture of audit and regulation, about the apparent decline in social cohesion and civility, about the threat of bioterrorism and war, at least you could take a stand on the issue of MMR. Although it may be irrational in scientific terms, the appeal of the option for separate vaccines is that it offers a 'third way' compromise between acceptance and outright rejection of the triple vaccine.

The MMR controversy provided a new opportunity for the assertion of rights in the sphere of health. If the assertion of a right confers no benefit on the person claiming it, and imposes no obligation on the agency to which the demand is addressed, it is likely to enjoy the enthusiastic support of middle-class activists and the media. The problem with the demand for the right to choose separate vaccines was that it could not be reconciled with the mass childhood immunisation campaign. Although the government's instinct (accurately reflected in the Prime Minister's household) was to indulge this demand, wiser counsels forbade this opportunist course. Thus, those insisting on their right to impose an inferior product and higher risks on their own children, were obliged to pursue this through the seedy private clinics that sprang up to meet this demand.

The focus of middle-class animosities on the MMR vaccine has a somewhat arbitrary character. Why immunisation? Few medical interventions over the second half of the twentieth century can compete with the record of safety and efficacy of vaccines. The balance of benefit to risk is much more questionable in relation to many other public health initiatives, notably cancer screening and the promotion of a healthy lifestyle, which retain popular approval (the fact that GPs also receive incentive payments for these activities is uncontroversial) (Fitzpatrick 2001). Why MMR? Of all the vaccines currently available, it has one of the lowest profiles of serious adverse reactions. Yet, in the peculiar constellation of circumstances that prevailed in Britain at the turn of the millennium, a scare about MMR captured the imagination of the fearful middle classes. This was unfortunate for those children who have missed MMR and are now at increased risk of these diseases; it was also unfortunate for children with autism, whose families were revisited with guilt and dragged into a futile quest for compensation through the courts.

# 5

# AUTISM AND PARENTS

'I'm going to ask everyone a question', said the conference host after Wakefield's talk. 'How many of you believe your children have been damaged by vaccines?'

Seventy-five per cent of the attendees stood up and raised their hands. One woman a few rows behind me was crying, and I knew intuitively that her faith in the medical establishment had finally crumbled. Her suffering was genuine; she sobbed quietly. When I looked back, she was embarrassed, covering her face with her hand.

But I was moved by her anguish, her private suffering, and I relived for a moment my own struggles since Connor's diagnosis. The long nights of guilt I felt as a mother, constantly wondering what I done wrong to give him autism; the long days of research to find a cure – the doctors told me to put him in an institution, but I wasn't going to leave him; the countless doctor visits and tests Connor bravely endured without understanding why he was hurting or receiving little relief.

And finally – unsurprisingly – I was overwhelmed with rage. I felt it building within me and it was like nothing I'd experienced before. I knew very clearly at that moment that I had crossed over to the other side, that I was convinced my son was a cash cow for an industry that tested its products in production rather than the lab, motivated by $2 billion per year in profits, no different in its potential for corruption that any other industry.

(Mitchell 2000: 1)

Lesli Mitchell's poignant testimony (following an address by Dr Wakefield to a conference in the USA in Spring 2000) captures the experience of many parents of autistic children who have become involved in the campaign against MMR. She articulates the deep distress felt by parents; the feelings of guilt and anger; the frustration over the inadequacies of medical investigation and treatment; the bitterness arising from contacts with insensitive doctors and other professionals. She also describes the cathartic effect of Dr Wakefield in transforming suppressed grief into outspoken rage and resentment, focused on vaccines and directed against the medical profession and the pharmaceutical corporations.

Although Lesli Mitchell presents her 'crossing over to the other side' as a process of enlightenment, it is important to recognise that, for all Dr Wakefield's undoubted charisma, his theory that MMR causes autism has not been substantiated. Nevertheless he currently continues to offer vaccines as a ready explanation for our children's difficulties and the drug companies as a convenient target for our sense of grievance – arguments which find an immediate resonance among parents of autistic children. The result is a climate of blame and recrimination, in which parents are ranged against doctors and other professionals and theories of conspiracy and corruption flourish as explanations for the relationships between the medical establishment, governments and drug companies.

In this chapter, I want to set the role of parents in the campaign against MMR in the wider context of evolving theories of autism since the condition was first recognised in the 1940s. I begin with my own experience as a parent, with some reflections on how this experience has been shaped by the changing understanding of autism in recent years. After a brief review of the conceptual framework for understanding and diagnosing autism that emerged in the 1980s, we then turn to look at two controversies that have raged among parents alongside the MMR story in the 1990s: the issues of 'regressive autism' and the 'autism epidemic'.

## A life sentence

Autism:

This neurodevelopmental disorder is, if severe, the antithesis of all that defines mental health.

Prevalence: up to 90/10,000 of those <16yrs old – estimates vary considerably. Sex ratio: M/F =3.

Autism is a triad of:

1. Impaired reciprocal social interaction (A symptoms).
2. Impaired imagination, associated with abnormal verbal and non-verbal communication (B symptoms).
3. Restricted repertoires of activities and interests (C symptoms).

Causes: (mostly unknown) prenatal rubella, tuberous sclerosis. MRI has shown neo-cerebellar hypoplasia (vermal lobules VI and VII).

Treatment: this is not effective. Behaviour therapy may be tried. *A good teacher is more helpful than a good doctor.*

70% remain severely handicapped. 50% will develop useful speech. 20% will develop seizures in adolescence. 15% will lead an independent life.

Apply for benefits (disability living allowance if in UK).
(Collier et al, 1997: 402)

The above text is from the *Oxford Handbook of Clinical Specialities*, which is a pocket-sized guide to diagnosis and treatment, popular with generations of junior hospital doctors. Its summary of medical wisdom on autism conveys with brutal economy the simple facts that doctors do not know what causes autism and have no treatment for it. Furthermore, the prognosis is grim: 'apply for benefits'.

'A lifelong disability: live with it' – this is the message that parents of autistic children have received from the medical profession. Some have had the bad news broken gently and sympathetically; some have had it delivered with all the sensitivity of the *Oxford Handbook*. In some ways, it makes little difference. You still have to find your own way of living with your child's strange behaviour, try to find ways of helping them, struggle to get them an education appropriate to their needs. You still have the eternal worry: what will become of our children when we are no longer around, or no longer able to look out for them?

As many doctors' spouses and children can testify, having a doctor in the family when somebody falls ill is often a mixed blessing. (When it comes to diagnosing and treating their own illnesses, doctors have an even worse reputation.) When, as a doctor, you realise that your son is autistic, there can be no delaying or softening of the impact of the bleak realities summarised in the *Oxford Handbook*. It falls like a hammer blow creating a feeling of utter impotence. If your children have ear infections or tonsillitis, or fall and cut their knees, you can at least make some practical suggestions. When the diagnosis is autism, you feel that all you can do is pass on counsels of despair.

There were however some advantages for us in my being a doctor. One was that we did not have to endure the shock of somebody else telling us the diagnosis. By the time we took James to our GP, we had already ticked the following features from the checklist of A, B and C symptoms as listed in the *Oxford Handbook* (I still have the sheet of paper):

A symptoms:

- marked unawareness of the existence and feelings of others
- abnormal response to being hurt
- impaired imitation
- abnormal play
- gross impairment in making peer friendships

B symptoms:

- no babbling, facial expressions or gestures
- avoids mutual gaze
- does not act adult roles

C symptoms:

- stereotyped movements
- preoccupation with parts of objects

Given that the diagnosis only requires two A symptoms, one B symptom and one C symptom, this can be considered almost the equivalent of an autistic spectrum full-house. Our GP was suitably sympathetic, and, no doubt, grateful that we had completed the diagnostic schedule. She immediately agreed to refer us to a local specialist clinic for further assessment. James was four weeks short of his second birthday.

Many parents of autistic children complain that they were often ill in infancy and had frequent courses of antibiotics for ear and other infections. This was not the case with James: he had only seen our GP once before he was diagnosed as autistic (with a viral illness). This was not because I had been diagnosing and treating him myself (I hadn't), but because he had always been remarkably healthy (indeed, this has continued). Although nobody thought this of any particular significance at the time, he had a full course of childhood immunisations, including MMR at about 14 months, without apparent misadventure.

It was still several months before we succeeded in getting official confirmation of the diagnosis of autism, following assessment at our local child development clinic. This was a grim period of anxiously watching and waiting, of hoping that James would somehow re-engage with us and the rest of the world, and of fearing that he might retreat still further. It was also a difficult time of deciding who to tell our sad news, and when and how to tell it. Of course, most of our close family and friends had already recognised the problem, even if they had not precisely named it. It was a relief when we could finally come out and tell them. Our problem was in finding ways of acknowledging James' diagnosis and of beginning to live our lives in full recognition of its consequences[1].

## Guilt and blame

Lesli Mitchell's recollection of 'long nights of guilt I felt as a mother, constantly wondering what I'd done wrong to give him autism' (Mitchell 2000) is one that strikes a chord with parents of autistic children. Most parents blame themselves for conditions suffered by their children: this tendency is particularly strong when the condition is apparent at birth or in early infancy, particularly when the cause of the condition is not understood. As a doctor, I have had discussions with mothers who have reviewed in detail their whole experience of pregnancy in the hope of discovering 'what they had done wrong' to explain some congenital abnormality. In the past such

---

1   One advantage of being a doctor was that I was able to attend a 'conference for professionals' organised by the National Autistic Society in London. Run by some of the leading British authorities on autism, this provided a high-level introduction. I left feeling much the wiser about autism and with a great respect for the National Autistic Society – a respect which has not diminished over subsequent years.

speculations have had a significant influence on medicine. Until the mid-twentieth century the notion that Down's syndrome resulted from excessive alcohol consumption during pregnancy was widely accepted by doctors (maternal denials were considered to only confirm that they drank in secret). The identification in 1959 of a chromosomal disorder (trisomy 21) as the cause of Down's syndrome banished the myth of the drunken mother (and some 39 other theories), but also signified the emergence of modern genetics and a more subtle conception of parental responsibility.

The long-running debate over the rival influences of nature and nurture, genes and environment, in normal development and in disease has raged in the world of autism since it was first identified, by the psychiatrist Leo Kanner in Baltimore in 1943. (There are several excellent accounts of the evolution of the concepts of autism over the past half-century, on which this brief summary is based [see Wing 1996, Frith 1989, 1991, Jordan 1999]. For contrasting psychological perspectives see Baron Cohen 1995, Hobson 2002.)

Kanner's historic paper opened with the statement that 'since 1938 there have come to our attention a number of children whose condition differs so markedly and uniquely from anything reported so far, that each case merits – and, I hope, will eventually receive – a detailed consideration of its fascinating peculiarities' (quoted in Frith 1989: 8). Kanner took over the term 'autistic' (from the Greek *autos*, meaning 'self'), which had first been used by the German psychiatrist Eugen Bleuler in 1911 to describe the characteristic withdrawal from social life of schizophrenics. Although Bleuler wrote of 'the detachment from reality, together with the relative and absolute preponderance of inner life' in schizophrenia, Kanner recognised the distinctive fact that autistic children had failed to enter the world in the first place and were 'strangers from the beginning'. In 1944 Hans Asperger, working in Austria, independently described a group of children with a similar condition, using the term 'autistic psychopathy'(Asperger 1991). (Because his paper was written in German during wartime, it did not become widely known in the English-speaking world until the 1980s.)

From his detailed case studies, Kanner emphasised two cardinal features of what he labelled 'early infantile autism'. The first was 'autistic aloneness' – the profound lack of emotional contact with other people these children displayed. The second was an obsessive insistence on sameness, manifested in repetitive movements and routines or a narrow range of interests. Asperger described children who never seemed to be 'on the same wavelength as their normal peers in any group activity'.

Kanner's much-quoted formulation that 'these children have come into the world with innate inability to form the usual, biologically-provided affective contact with people' indicates two key convictions (quoted in Frith 1989: 9). He believed that the core deficit in autism lay in the capacity to establish emotional (affective) relationships. He also believed that this was 'innate' or 'biologically-provided': that autism resulted from some, as yet unidentified, disorder of anatomy or physiology present in these children from birth. Asperger, who studied the families of some 200 children over a ten-year period, was even more explicit in his belief that autism was a constitutional or genetic disorder: 'from the second year of life we find already the characteristic features which remain unmistakable and constant throughout the whole lifespan' (Asperger 1991: 67).

Both Kanner and Asperger commented on what they regarded as distinctive features of the parents of autistic children. Kanner noted that they tended to be highly intelligent, well educated and of high occupational status. He also found them to be 'cold, bookish, formal, introverted, disdainful of frivolity, humourless, detached and highly – even excessively – rational and objective' (quoted in Rimland 1965: 30). Asperger observed that 'in every single case where it was possible to make a closer acquaintance' with the family of an autistic child, it was the father who appeared to 'have transmitted the autistic traits' (Asperger 1991: 84). Like Kanner, he noted that fathers tended 'to occupy high social positions', despite their 'noticeable peculiarities'. Both commented on the prevalence of the stereotype of the 'absent-minded professor' among autistic families.

Although in his original paper Kanner implied that the significance of parental personality lay in the probable inheritance of autistic features, his outlook shifted over the next 20 years under the influence of the dominant Freudian psychoanalytic tradition in American psychiatry. From this perspective, the origins of most psychiatric disorders could be discovered in early infantile experience, particularly in difficulties in child–parent relationships. Just as severe mental illness in adults was blamed on the 'schizophrenogenic mother', autism was attributed to defective parenting. According to this 'psychogenic' theory, expounded by Kanner in a notorious interview in *Time Magazine* in 1960, autistic children were 'the offspring of highly organised professional parents' who 'just happened to defrost long enough to produce a child' – a child who 'was not really wanted' (quoted in Rimland 1965: 32). The 'refrigerator mother', whose coldness drove her baby into autistic withdrawal, provided a popular explanation for this obscure condition. Although the psychogenic theory has long been discredited, this cruel metaphor and the prejudice it expresses have continued to haunt parents of autistic children.

The psychogenic theory of autism was popularised by Bruno Bettelheim, whose 1967 book *The Empty Fortress* – a collection of essays subtitled 'infantile autism and the birth of the self' – is still in print (Bettelheim 1967). His central argument, which derived particular authority from his own experience of incarceration in a Nazi concentration camp, was that autistic children were, like prisoners in the camps who adopted an autistic-like state of withdrawal, reacting to 'an extreme situation'. He postulated that the initial cause of autistic withdrawal was 'the child's correct interpretation of the negative emotions with which the most significant figures in his environment approach him' (Bettelheim 1967: 66). For Bettelheim, autism was 'a state of mind that develops in reaction to feeling oneself in an extreme situation, entirely without hope' (Bettelheim 1967: 68). He recommended that children be removed from their parents to specialised institutional care where they could receive intensive psychotherapy.

As numerous commentators have pointed out, there was no evidence for the psychogenic theory. It was based on an analogy between an autistic child and a concentration camp victim, which was plausible and compelling, particularly given the proximity of the experience of the Holocaust personified by Bettelheim himself. But the theory was speculative and false. Furthermore, by explicitly blaming parents it compounded the suffering arising from having an autistic child, causing family separation and, in some cases, marital breakdown. It has left a legacy of distrust for any aspect of the psychodynamic tradition among autism parents.

One reason for the enduring influence of Bettelheim's work is that his approach implied a therapeutic optimism that the alternative 'constitutional' theory implicitly denied (although Bettelheim's career has received a highly critical evaluation in Richard Pollack's biography (Pollack 1996); see also Dineen 1999). He argued that if autism was regarded as an 'inborn impairment', the 'resultant attitudes towards treatment will be defeatist' (Bettelheim 1967: 405). On the other hand, those who 'trace the causes of autism at least in part to the environmental influence' tend to be 'more optimistic', because of 'the not always valid, but convincing belief that what environment has caused, environment may also be able to correct'. This outlook is still influential among parents today.

In the course of the 1960s and 1970s, parents played a significant role in challenging the dominant psychogenic school on both sides of the Atlantic. It is striking that they did this through working and writing in a professional capacity – as psychologists and psychiatrists – rather than as parents of autistic children. Their efforts proved influential in bringing together parents and professionals in the first autism organisations. Key figures were Dr Bernard Rimland (a psychologist) in the USA and Drs Lorna and John Wing (both psychiatrists) in Britain (although both Rimland and the Wings had autistic children, this was not mentioned in their early publications).

Bernard Rimland's 1965 book *Infantile Autism: The syndrome and its implications for a neural theory of behavior*, written while he was working as a psychologist in the US navy, directly challenged the psychogenic theory (Rimland 1965). Noting the plausibility of this approach, Dr Rimland argued that it had been 'accepted without evaluation or evidence' and insisted that the fact that many parents exhibited distinctive personality features was more suggestive of a biological than a psychological cause. He pointed out that some parents did not conform to the now familiar stereotype (though he suggested that only a meagre 10 per cent were 'warm and friendly'). Although he was keen to remove parents from blame, Dr Rimland upheld Kanner's conviction that they were of superior intellect, suggesting that autistic children were genetically vulnerable as a consequence of an 'unborn capacity for high intelligence' – his 'brightness gone awry hypothesis'.

Taking the case for biological causation together with the lack of evidence for psychogenic causation, Dr Rimland concluded that it was difficult to understand the continuing popularity of the latter approach, especially given what he described as its 'pernicious implications':

> To add a heavy burden of shame and guilt to the distress of people whose hopes, social life, finances, well-being and feelings of worth have been all but destroyed seems heartless and inconsiderate in the extreme.
>
> (Rimland, 1965: 65)

Dr Rimland's book became a powerful weapon in the hands of parents challenging the baleful influence of parent-blaming theories, especially in the USA, where they were more influential than in

Britain. (While Dr Rimland led the campaign against the psychogenic theory in the USA, it had already been challenged by Dr Mildred Creak, child psychiatrist at Great Ormond Street Hospital in London, and others, in the late 1950s and early 1960s.) Dr Rimland played a leading role in forming the first autism advocacy group in the USA and he remains a prominent activist.

Dr Rimland also suggested that autism might be a result of a specific cognitive dysfunction – a 'grossly impaired ability to relate new stimuli to remembered experience' – which arose from a defect in a particular area of the brain known as the reticular formation. The problem with these neurological hypotheses is that they were every bit as speculative as the psychogenic theory. They were also vulnerable to the riposte that they did not suggest any specific therapeutic intervention.

Published in 1966, *Early Childhood Autism: Clinical, educational and social aspects* (Wing, J.K. 1966) brought together contributions from a number of pioneers in the emerging field of autism in Britain. These included his wife Lorna Wing, Michael Rutter (subsequently Britain's leading child psychiatrist), Beate Hermelin (famous for her later researches into the psychology of autism, mainly conducted jointly with Neil O'Connor) and Victor Lotter (the psychiatrist who conducted the first epidemiological study of autism). The practical thrust of the book was reflected in chapters from Ivar Lovaas (pioneer of the 'applied behaviour analysis' teaching method) and Sybil Elgar (head of the first dedicated school for autistic children in London). Margaret Lauder contributed a chapter from a parent's perspective. The multidisciplinary character of the book and its combination of theoretical discussion with a strongly practical orientation towards 'what works' for autistic children reflected the more pragmatic approach to the subject that has prevailed in Britain.

The British authorities were briskly dismissive of the psychogenic theory and emphasised that 'no case has been made that psychoanalysis or a psychoanalytic orientation has any specific effect in the treatment of autistic children' (Connell 1966: 109). Chapters by Rutter and Hermelin indicated the growing interest in exploring the links between cognitive and affective deficits in autistic children. The contributors expressed an acute recognition of the distress experienced by families affected by autism, often compounded by the prejudices held by professionals as well as the general public. Lorna Wing commented that 'by the time parents come round to seeking expert help they are usually unhappy, bewildered, guilt-ridden and completely without confidence in their own child' (Wing, L. 1966:

260). In other chapters, authors with experience of dealing with autistic children indicated ways in which behavioural problems could be overcome and how children could be helped to learn.

## A disorder of development

Since the 1980s the concept of autism as a disorder of development has become widely accepted. A consensus has emerged among scientists, doctors and parents that autism results from some defect in the structure or function of the brain. Although the nature and causes of this defect remain obscure, research and clinical work in a number of areas have contributed to a deepening understanding of the range of features characteristic of autism.

The recognition that autism is linked with conditions in which some form of brain damage is a recognised feature provides important support for the biological theory of autism. Psychometric testing, including IQ tests, reveals that up to one third of autistic children fall into the range of mental handicap (or 'severe learning difficulty'), and in two-thirds the IQ is below average. Around 30 per cent of autistic children develop epileptic fits in adolescence, if not earlier. Children with a range of genetic conditions (Fragile X, tuberous sclerosis, neurofibromatosis) are at increased risk of becoming autistic. Autism may also result from viral infections, such as rubella and cytomegalovirus, affecting the fetus during pregnancy, and from herpes encephalitis in babies (although neither rubella nor measles have been shown to cause autism in children). Autism has also been associated with a number of rare metabolic and congenital abnormality syndromes. This range of conditions accounts for around 10 per cent of cases of autism, but in the large majority no such cause of brain damage can be identified.

Twin and family studies have provided growing support for a substantial genetic contribution to autism (Bailey et al 1995, Bolton, Rutter 2001). If twins are identical and one is diagnosed as autistic, the chances that the other will also be autistic are around 60 per cent; the chances of having some autistic spectrum disorder are up to 90 per cent. If they are non-identical, the risk is similar to that of other siblings, around 6 per cent for autism, but up to 20 per cent for some form of autistic disorder (the risk in the general population is less than 1 per cent). However, the fact that in 10 per cent or more of cases involving identical twins only one twin becomes autistic, confirms that some additional factor or factors, probably acting at an early stage of fetal development, play a part in causing the damage that results in autism. In the course of the 1990s research in genetics identified a number of genes that appear to be important in the genesis of autism. Wider family studies have suggested that a susceptibility to autism may be associated with a vulnerability to learning difficulties and other psychological problems in close relatives.

Epidemiological studies have revealed a number of characteristics of autism that are difficult to reconcile with the psychogenic theory. As any visit to a school for autistic children immediately confirms, the condition is much more common among boys, by a proportion of four or five to one. Among 'higher-functioning' children and those with Asperger's syndrome, the male excess is even higher; at lower levels of intelligence, the gender balance is more even. Contrary to the impressions of early observers (who tended to be American psychiatrists in private practice), large-scale studies confirm that autism can be found, at comparable rates, among all social classes and ethnic groups. It also appears to occur at similar rates in different countries and different cultures.

Perhaps the most disappointing area of research into autism has been in the field of neuroscience. In the late 1980s Eric Courchesne and colleagues in the USA created great excitement when they identified abnormalities of the cerebellum (detailed in the summary in the *Oxford Handbook* quoted above) as the possible root cause of autism. But these findings, and numerous subsequent claims for the role of particular brain regions or neurotransmitters, resulting from a wide range of scanning and biochemical techniques, have not been confirmed. Despite a long and intensive quest, the underlying 'final common pathway' in the human brain, through which a range of genetic and environmental factors result in autism, remains elusive.

The study of autistic children led to the formulation of two concepts that have had a major impact on the understanding of autism. These are the characterisation of a *triad* of impairments as the core features of autism and the notion of autism as a *spectrum* of related conditions.

Based on their epidemiological study in the old south London borough of Camberwell in the 1970s, Lorna Wing and Judith Gould identified three clusters of features that they considered diagnostic of autism (Wing 1996). The characteristic impairments were in *social interaction* (many children were aloof and indifferent to others, some were passive, others were 'active but odd'); in *communication* (many children had no language, in others language was deviant, repetitive, stereotypical or limited to 'echoing' others); in *imagination* (children were unable to engage in 'pretend play', others displayed rigidity of thought and behaviour, following rituals and routines). This framework reflected a more precise understanding of the behaviour of autistic children and facilitated the emergence of clearer diagnostic criteria. It also led to a growing recognition of the different features of autism in children at different levels of cognitive ability and at different ages and stages of development. Thus, although they shared the core features of the triad, autistic individuals might manifest quite different forms of behaviour, and experience different problems.

One of the consequences of using the 'triad of impairments' as a set of diagnostic criteria was the inclusion of a much larger number of children within the label of autism. It particularly led to an increased number of diagnoses of autism at both ends of the range of cognitive abilities: among those formerly classified as 'mentally handicapped' or 'mentally retarded', and among those with an IQ that was in the normal range or above average, but who manifested the typical picture of what came to be known as 'Asperger's syndrome' (Frith 1991). Children with Asperger's are stilted in social interaction and appear lacking in empathy. They tend to have pedantic and stereotyped speech and impaired non-verbal communication. They often have circumscribed interests (occasionally having specialised skills in mathematics, music or other areas) and are physically clumsy. The triad thus led to the concept of autism as a 'continuum' or 'spectrum' of disorders, in which the presentation of individuals varied according to the extent of their social and intellectual impairments.

Together with the mounting evidence for the biological origins of the condition, the diagnostic triad helped to establish the distinctive nature of autism with respect to other conditions in the field of child psychiatry. Many children who until the 1980s would have been diagnosed as 'psychotic' or 'schizophrenic', or as having a 'schizoid personality disorder', would now be diagnosed as autistic. Schizophrenia, which rarely appears before adolescence, is now never diagnosed in young children; the distinction is also strengthened by the recognition that it is very rare for autistic children to develop schizophrenia in later life. The sharper focus on impairments of social interaction and communication in autism also helped to clarify the distinction between this condition and the wider range of mental disabilities.

Parents generally welcomed both the clearer understanding of the condition affecting their children and the wider recognition of this disorder among doctors, psychiatrists and teachers. The definition of autism as a disorder of development rather than as a psychiatric condition like schizophrenia has meant that parents have been able to avoid some of the stigma associated with mental illness, as well as helping put an end to 'parent-blaming'. The concept of autism as a spectrum of disorders also helped to reduce the distance between children with autism and 'normal' children. Increasing professional – and public – understanding of Asperger's syndrome led to the recognition that some of the features of autism, such as a lack of social skills or empathy, unusual patterns of speech and obsessive and ritualistic behaviours could be identified in many people (particularly males).

The success of the film *Rain Man*, for which Dustin Hoffman won an Oscar in 1989 for his depiction of a man with autism (who also had certain 'savant' mathematical skills), did much to raise popular awareness. It also led to a popular over-estimation of the frequency with which such skills occur among people with autism. In fact they are quite rare, and often coexist with other impairments, which mean that the skills have little practical value.

On the other hand, the tendency to label as autistic every absent-minded professor and eccentric scientist, and every obsessive engineer, train-spotter and stamp-collector (compounded by the vogue for identifying historical figures and even contemporary celebrities as autistic) carries the risk that the spectrum becomes stretched so wide that autism loses its distinctiveness. 'Normalising' autism may reduce stigma, but at the cost of diminishing recognition of the extreme aloneness that results from the social impairment of autism, even in higher functioning individuals. Temple Grandin is a professor of veterinary science at Colorado State University and the title of Oliver Sacks' account of her life (Sacks 1995) – *An Anthropologist on Mars* – is Grandin's own description of what she feels like when trying to engage with other people, and clearly expresses the profound sense of alienation experienced by even the highest-functioning people with autism.

## 'Regressive' autism

Campaigners against MMR have argued that a new and distinctive form of autism, characterised as 'regressive', has emerged as a result of the effects of the MMR vaccine. It is claimed that 'regressive' autism is distinguished by a sudden loss of skills and deterioration in behaviour following the MMR immunisation, after a prior period of normal development.

When I first heard rumours of a link between MMR and autism, I dug out James' old baby clinic record-book to check the dates. Sure enough he had the MMR when he was 14 months old, about four months before we first became concerned about him and six months before we first recognised that he might be autistic. We had no recollection of any adverse reaction at the time. I vividly recall a paediatrician who saw James some months later, summarising our account, saying 'So, you felt he was completely normal up to about 18 months?' 'Normal', I thought to myself did not begin to describe how wonderful he was: like any happy, playful toddler. (Nor was he, like some babies who are later diagnosed as autistic, abnormally quiet and passive; his brother was only 16 months older so we were quite familiar with normal patterns of development.) When James first became withdrawn and avoided eye contact, our first thought was that something might have happened to him. At the time we never considered MMR, and in retrospect it seemed a remote event, difficult to relate to his insidious decline, although it is understandable that other parents, for whom the event was more closely related to a more precipitous decline, might make some connection. Watching an apparently 'normal' – wonderful – child regress into the detached and disturbed behaviours of autism is a traumatic experience for parents, and anybody who can offer a plausible explanation is likely to get a hearing.

However, although this pattern of regression was unfamiliar to us – as it is to most other parents – it has been recognised by researchers into autism for decades, long before MMR was introduced. While in the majority of children diagnosed as autistic, problems become apparent within the first 12 months, in a substantial minority a period of apparently normal development continues up to 15 or 18 months, which is then followed by a loss of skills and a deterioration of behaviour (in the very period when MMR is usually given). Rates of regression or loss of skills ranging from 20 to 50 per cent have been reported in both epidemiological and clinical samples (Fombonne, Chakrabarti, 2001). In their comparative study, Fombonne and Chakrabarti found that children with a history of regression had no other developmental or clinical characteristics that distinguished them from other children with autism. In these children it is usually possible in retrospect to recognise that abnormal features were present before regression became apparent, although their significance may not have been recognised by parents or even by professionals. (For example, children may not have pointed to show things to others or have played 'peek-a-boo' or 'hide-and-seek'. This was true of James.) It may also be the case that whatever language children have developed is limited and repetitive (often simply 'echoing' others) and that their skills are isolated and do not reflect any growing understanding of the world[2]. Another confusion has arisen in relation to childhood disintegrative disorder (CDD) (Wing, Potter 2002). In this, very rare, condition the child develops normally up to the age of at least 2 years, more commonly beyond 3, when there is a dramatic loss of language, social skills and adaptive behaviour, accompanied by loss of continence and motor abnormalities. Although there may be some difficulty in distinguishing this condition from childhood autism, the recognition of earlier developmental abnormalities in autism and the later and more drastic loss of cognitive skills in CDD usually clarify the diagnosis[3].

Dr Wakefield states that 'in children with regressive autism, the emerging behavioural phenotype is of regression in a previously developmentally normal child' (Wakefield 1999: 1). This is, as discussed above, not an 'emerging' phenomenon, but the familiar pattern in a substantial minority of cases. However, Dr Wakefield continues, 'this is consistent with an early-onset disintegrative disorder in which contact with reality and communication disintegrates after previously normal development'. Here Dr Wakefield seems to confuse childhood autism (which in many cases first presents with features of regression) with the distinctive pattern of CDD.

The lack of precision in characterising the 'regression' in cases of autism which have been attributed to MMR has caused some exasperation among autism experts (Fombonne 2001). Dr Lorna Wing is

---

2  A Checklist for Autism in Toddlers (CHAT) using questions like this has been developed for screening children for autism at 18 months (Baird et al 2000, Baron Cohen et al 2000).

3  The series of 12 cases presented by Dr Wakefield in his February 1998 *Lancet* paper includes one in which CDD was suspected (Wakefield 1998). His expanded series of 60 cases presented two years later includes two cases of CDD (Wakefield 2000). However, this suggests a prevalence of CDD in his series (3.3%) much higher than the rate of 1.7 cases per 10,000 (0.017%) that Fombonne estimates from the four surveys in different countries that have attempted to quantify this condition (Fombonne 2002). As Fombonne indicates, this 'raises the possibility that CDD might be a component of the phenotype of the hypothesised MMR-induced autism'. However, he found no evidence for a link between MMR and CDD and no evidence for an increase in rates of CDD.

quoted in one account as saying that she 'did not believe in the existence of regressive autism' (Wing 2001). She distinguished carefully between the regression that occurs in the very small number of cases of CDD and the familiar loss of skills in children with autism at some time in the second year.

## The autism epidemic

'The autism world is in crisis, with the number of children affected skyrocketing' declared Dr Wakefield on his departure from the Royal Free (Wakefield 2001a). Claims of an explosion of autism became a recurrent theme in the statements of anti-MMR activists and have also featured prominently in the popular press. These claims are supported by a wide range of anecdotes telling of dramatic increases in numbers of cases, reflected in demands for special services, pressures on schools, membership of local autism organisations. Numerous surveys also indicate an increased rate of diagnosis in communities from Surrey to California.

For parents who may have known little about autism before their child's diagnosis, the idea of an 'autism epidemic' rings true. They generally grew up in the 1960s and 1970s when there was little public recognition of autism; they had children in the 1980s and 1990s when awareness grew steadily. Parents of children with autism soon meet other local parents with autistic children. Having lived for 20 or 30 years without ever knowing an individual or family affected by autism, suddenly they know many, perhaps within the same community in which they have always lived. Parents naturally draw the conclusion that their perception of an increased number of people with autism reflects a real increase.

The 'autism epidemic' has become an article of faith for the anti-MMR campaign. Not only does it correspond to parents' experience, it provides intuitive confirmation of an environmental cause for autism (such as vaccination). The dominant orthodox medical theory, that attributes autism largely to genetic causes, cannot explain a rapid increase in the number of cases over a relatively short period of time. But is there really an epidemic of autism?

Whereas for commentators with little experience in the epidemiology of autism, the epidemic appears to be a straightforward fact, experts in the field are much more circumspect. When asked about the 'huge percentage increases being noted over the last ten years in the USA', in an interview for the 'Autism99' Internet conference, the neurologist and author Oliver Sacks drew a parallel with his experience of Tourette's syndrome (Sacks 1999). He noted that in the 1960s and 1970s Tourette's was considered very rare, but after he became interested in the subject, he began to recognise more and more cases just walking on the streets in New York. After seeing five people in two days, he thought to himself 'this must be a thousand times commoner' than he had thought. On reflection, he decided that 'it has not become commoner, we've simply become more aware of it'. Dr Sacks suspected that 'something of the sort may be the case with autism'. He recalled that, until quite recently, autism 'wasn't recognised or talked about'. When he worked in a state mental hospital in the 1970s, 'people with autism were not clearly differentiated from people with retardation or people with schizophrenia or other conditions'. How did he explain the autism epidemic? 'I think it's probably our clearer perception of what constitutes autism'.

The question of whether autism is becoming more common has been a matter of some controversy among experts for more than a decade (Gillberg et al 1991). In a review of the literature published two years before Dr Wakefield's *Lancet* paper, Dr Lorna Wing discussed the formidable difficulties in making a definitive judgement (Wing 1996). In particular, she pointed to the paucity and poor quality of data and the problems of case definition and improvements in diagnosis. Her agnostic conclusion was that there was 'no evidence for or against an increase in prevalence'. Reviewing 23 epidemiological studies of autism in 1999, Dr Eric Fombonne noted a significant increase in prevalence in the decade following 1988 compared with the two decades preceding this date (Fombonne 1999). However, he attributed this increase to changes in case definition and improved recognition.

In a further study published in 2001, Fombonne and Chakrabarti came to the conclusion that the discovery of higher rates in recent surveys 'merely reflects the adoption of a much broader concept of autism, a recognition of autism among normally intelligent subjects and an improved identification of persons with autism' (Fombonne, Chakrabarti 2001). Dr Fombonne particularly dismissed a survey from California, widely cited by proponents of an epidemic, as being statistically flawed. His hard-hitting conclusion was that there was 'no need to raise false alarms of putative epidemics, nor to practice poor science to draw attention to the unmet needs of large numbers of seriously impaired adults and children' (Fombonne 2001: 413). Another study has noted that the increase in the number of cases identified with autism in California almost exactly equals the decline in the number of cases identified as having 'mental retardation'. The authors concluded that 'improvements in detection and changes in diagnosis account for the observed increase in autism; whether there has also been a true increase in incidence is not known' (Croen et al 2002: 207).

Why is it so difficult to judge whether autism is on the rise? It is important to recall that until recently autism was regarded as a rare, even 'very rare', condition and there is still no official register of cases. Estimates of numbers thus rely on local studies, conducted at different times, in different places, often with different objectives and using different methods and different diagnostic categories. Such studies are also of different sizes and of variable quality, all factors affecting how far their conclusions can be reliably generalised. There is no definitive test for autism: the diagnosis rests on a clinical judgement of behaviour. In the past most studies investigated the *prevalence* of autism – the number of cases in a specified population at a particular time. Some recent studies have investigated the *incidence* of autism – the number of new cases identified in a given population over a given time period, usually 12 months. These approaches have distinct advantages and difficulties.

Studies of prevalence are most appropriate for identifying people with a chronic condition, particularly for purposes of planning services. Their accuracy is influenced by the size of the target population and by the rigour of the methods that are used to identify cases. The results may also be affected by the social characteristics of the population, by factors such as social class, ethnicity, rates of immigration and emigration. Another important factor is whether the study seeks to identify autistic children from the full range of ability (some early studies excluded either children with very low IQ or those with IQ in the normal range). Studies of incidence are most suitable for acute conditions, such as infectious diseases. The particular difficulty in relation to autism arises from the fact that its onset is often insidious and diagnosis is often delayed. Although parents may have recognised problems at an earlier stage, studies have tended to regard the year of diagnosis as the year of onset. As a result of the recent growth in awareness of autism, among both professionals and the public, there is a trend for earlier diagnosis, creating the appearance of a rising incidence.

A number of factors may have contributed to a rise in the numbers of diagnoses of autism (Wing, Potter 2002). First, changes in diagnostic criteria have expanded the range of diagnosis. Whereas early surveys focused on classical 'Kanner's' autism, the inclusion of children with Asperger's syndrome and those with atypical autism has inevitably boosted numbers. Second, there has been a growing recognition that autism could be found among both children with severe mental retardation and those with high intellectual ability. Third, the efforts of parents' organisations, clinicians and researchers have encouraged greater professional understanding of autism, while films, books and newspaper features have fostered a growing awareness of the condition among the public. Fourth, the decline of residential institutions and the rise of specialist provision for the care and education of children and adults with particular educational and other needs have helped to make the diagnosis of autism less stigmatising and more beneficial for parents.

Of course, the influence of these factors does not exclude the possibility that the rise in numbers of children with autism is a real increase, resulting from some new environmental cause. However, looking back on her own studies in Camberwell and those of Christopher Gillberg in Gothenburg, both carried out in the 1970s, Lorna Wing made an interesting observation (Wing, Potter 2002). In Camberwell, the study found the rate of children with autism with an IQ less than 70 was 20 in 10,000; the comparable rate in Gothenburg was 18 in 10,000. The Gothenberg study also found children with Asperger's syndrome at a rate of 35 in 10,000 and with atypical autism at 36 in 10,000. Adding the Gothenburg cases together gave an overall rate of autistic spectrum disorders of 89 in 10,000 – a figure similar to, if not higher than, rates found in recent studies. She reckoned that 'if the case finding had been as thorough and the same criteria for the whole autistic spectrum had been applied' the rates found would have been 'even higher than most of those found recently'.

In their comprehensive review of the epidemiology of autistic spectrum disorders, Wing and Potter came to the following conclusion:

> The evidence suggests that most, if not all, the reported rise in incidence and prevalence is due to changes in diagnostic criteria and increasing awareness and recognition of autistic spectrum disorders. Whether there is also a genuine rise in incidence remains an open question.
>
> (Wing, Potter 2002: 2)

# 6

# ALTERNATIVE AUTISM

The Defeat Autism Now! (DAN!) network (see below) summarises its 'current understanding of the biology of autism' in terms of the following 'inter-related factors':

- nutritional deficiencies and special needs – these concern primarily Vitamins B6, B12, A and magnesium, calcium, selenium, zinc, and omega 3 fatty acids;
- gut dysfunction due to multiple factors, including suboptimal nutrition, infections, antibiotics and non-steroidal anti-inflammatory drugs;
- microbial overgrowth including viral infections in susceptible children after a) certain vaccines, b) intestinal parasites, and c) bacterial and yeast overgrowths in the gut;
- toxins, such as PCBs, and particularly heavy metals, such as mercury from environmental sources and certain childhood vaccines;
- food intolerance, including intolerance of gluten and casein (found in grains and dairy), immunoglobulin-mediated food allergy (not always evident on skin-testing), intolerance of so-called Feingold foods and additives (phenolic compounds), and excitotoxins (certain flavour enhancers from the MSG family);
- abnormalities in detox chemistry and immune function;
- benefits from secretin, intravenous immunoglobulin (IVIG), transfer factor, colostrum, and special digestive enzymes in many individuals with autistic symptoms. (Rimland 2002)

When parents of an autistic child enquire about what sort of research is going on into the condition affecting their child, they may be told of exciting developments in genetics. But this is scant consolation. It reinforces feelings of guilt that 'it is something we passed on' and encourages recriminations about which side of the family may have contributed the defective genes. Worse, as Bettelheim and other psychoanalysts historically pointed out, genetic determinism invites therapeutic nihilism (see Chapter 5). If the problem is in the child's genes, then what can be done about it? Genetics may give clues towards prevention (even that seems a long way in the future) but it offers no help in the here and now, and it is in the here and now that parents of autistic children need help. Neither do ingenious experiments in cognitive psychology nor colourful images from the latest brain scanning devices offer practical solutions to our day-to-day difficulties.

Parents know that research takes time to yield results, but we cannot escape from the question of what is to be done – *now*. Parents' frustration at the lack of understanding of autism, and the absence of any definitive treatment drive the quest for alternative theories and therapies. Although these raise hopes and satisfy the need 'to do something', they tend to result in disappointment – and the costs may be high, perhaps in financial terms, but more importantly in depleting already strained reserves of energy and optimism and intensifying the pressures on the family.

The unorthodox biomedical approach summarised in the DAN! statement quoted above has become a major influence on parents on both sides of the Atlantic, and it is strongly held by many parents who blame MMR for their children's difficulties. Before looking at this approach in more detail, a brief survey at two earlier alternative approaches – holding therapy and secretin – may help to put current controversies in a wider context.

## Holding therapy

In the 1970s the Nobel Laureate Nikolaas Tinbergen and his wife Elisabeth, who had an autistic son, extended their 'ethological' studies of animals in their natural habitat to autistic children. They concluded that the origins of autistic behaviour lay in 'motivational conflict': the basic desire of the autistic child to approach others was offset by anxiety leading to avoidance of contact. They collaborated with the Oxford autism specialist John Richer, who observed that when adults intervened in an attempt to overcome the avoidance behaviour of autistic children, this tended to be counterproductive, making them withdraw further.

Martha Welch, an American psychiatrist, proposed 'holding therapy' as a method of overcoming motivational conflict, and it was taken up with enthusiasm by the Tinbergens and Richer. Here is a recent account of the 'holding therapy' process:

> The therapy . . . aimed at overcoming fear of emotional contact by close and sustained physical contact between the child and his/her mother, usually with the child sitting on the mother's lap and facing her. The role of the therapist was to help the mother initiate and maintain the hold, and to develop direct eye contact. As the child would typically find such close and prolonged contact disagreeable or frightening, considerable force was often needed to maintain it.
>
> (Roth 2002: 291)

This dramatic procedure provoked much controversy when it was shown in a BBC television documentary in 1988. Although many found it distressing to watch, its promoters claimed dramatic results: one 3-year-old was said to have progressed after six weeks' holding therapy from being 'mute, unable to relate to people, hyperactive, developmentally retarded' to being able to say words. By the age of 8 he was reported to be normal 'both intellectually and in his social relationships'. Indeed the Tinbergens' 1985 account of holding therapy was entitled *Autistic Children: New hope for a cure* (Tinbergen, Tinbergen 1985).

Critics noted that, for most autistic children, anxiety was not particularly associated with approach behaviour and disputed that adult intervention increased withdrawal. Indeed, some claimed that, on the contrary, it improved social interaction. When it came to explaining the origins of autism, the Tinbergens tended to resort to psychogenic factors such as early childhood trauma. When critics pointed out that most children who experienced early separation from their parents and institutional care did not become autistic, Richer argued that such experiences only induced autism in a small group with increased vulnerability as a result of constitutional factors. There were also difficulties in evaluating the claims made by holding therapy enthusiasts: there were uncertainties about the diagnosis of some of the children and unsatisfactory arrangements for assessment and follow-up.

While there was anecdotal evidence of success, there were also stories of failure. One mother found that three years of holding therapy

> led to us becoming locked in a situation of almost unbearable tension; spontaneity disappeared from our holding sessions as I increased my efforts to do what was required. I felt a failure, which in turn made me feel I must try harder. It was a vicious circle . . .

Holding therapy, she concluded 'can be damaging' (Hocking 1987). Therese Joliffe, an adult with autism, reflected bitterly on her experience of holding therapy as a child: 'to me the suffering was terrible and it achieved nothing' (Joliffe et al 1992).

After a brief period of popularity in the 1980s, holding therapy was abandoned in Britain. It remains controversial in the USA where it is still used to deal with children with behavioural problems (not specifically autistic children) despite attempts to have it banned as a form of child abuse.

## Secretin

Secretin is a hormone that stimulates the release of digestive juices from the pancreas, stomach and liver. It has no known therapeutic use, but as a preparation extracted from pig intestine it is (rarely) used to test whether the pancreas is functioning normally. It is not licensed as a treatment and, as a fairly crude pork product, carries a risk of provoking allergic reactions and other side effects (Kallen 1999a).

In the USA in 1996 Victoria Beck took her autistic son Parker Tucker for a gastrointestinal investigation, which involved an injection of secretin. Over the next three months she noticed a dramatic improvement in his autistic symptoms: he began speaking again, sleeping well and eating normally. Convinced that secretin had produced this improvement, she asked her doctors to continue prescribing it. In October 1998 Beck told her story on the *Dateline NBC* television show and provoked an immediate surge in demands for secretin from parents of autistic children. A study of her son and two other boys with autism, carried out by Dr Karoly Horvath, a Baltimore paediatrician, appeared to confirm the story: secretin was said to produce dramatic improvements in behaviour, particularly in eye contact and expressive language (Horvath et al 1999).

Thousands of parents sought out doctors who would agree to prescribe secretin 'off-licence' and carry out a course of intravenous infusions. As supplies were rapidly depleted, a black market emerged and prices rocketed.

The secretin story hit Britain in summer 1999, in the form of two episodes of the *Tonight with Trevor McDonald* news magazine programme. The show told 'Billy's Story' – how Billy Tommey, a little boy with autism, had shown a 'tremendous improvement' after receiving a course of secretin injections from a private GP in London. (The cost of this course of six injections was around £1,500. This GP also offers specialist anti-ageing preparations as well as treatment for jetlag, chronic fatigue syndrome and impotence.) 'Before' and 'after' film footage of Billy appeared to confirm the miraculous effect.

Secretin was enthusiastically endorsed by some prominent figures in the world of alternative autism. In the USA, Dr Bernard Rimland of the Autism Research Institute in San Diego, claimed, on the strength of testimonials he had received from 300 parents, that it was 'the most important development in the history of autism'. In Britain, Paul Shattock, a pharmacist and lecturer, father of an (adult) autistic son and director of the Autism Research Unit at the University of Sunderland, also endorsed secretin. Given the difficulties of securing supplies of secretin in Britain, Ainsworth's Homoeopathic Pharmacy marketed a 'homoeopathic secretin' product, which was endorsed by Mr Shattock.

The secretin bubble burst in December 1999, when a double-blind placebo-controlled trial of secretin in 60 autistic children concluded that it was not an effective treatment (Sandler et al 1999). Four further trials have echoed this conclusion. In an editorial accompanying the December 1999 study, the American autism authority Professor Fred Volkmar drew out some 'Lessons from Secretin':

> The extensive media attention when substantive supporting data were absent was clearly premature and unfortunate. Parents scrambled to obtain this 'cure' for their children in the absence of data on safety and efficacy – aided, in some cases, by well-meaning, if not well-informed, health care professionals. What makes an interesting television programme may not, of course, be the same as what makes good science.
>
> (Volkmar 1999: 1845)

Professor Volkmar emphasised the danger of relying on anecdotes and studies such as Horvath's:

Unfortunately, claims may be made on the basis of uncontrolled single-case reports with all the attendant problems (eg ambiguities regarding diagnosis and the nature of the treatment and the fact that some children improve without intervention).

His final words were for parents and their doctors:

Pursuing unproven treatments risks depleting the financial and psychosocial resources of families. It is important that physicians help families make informed decisions about treatment for autism.

(Volkmar 1999: 1845)

In autumn 1999, Jonathan and Polly Tommey, Billy's parents, launched *The Autism File* – a magazine promoting a range of alternative interventions, including secretin. In the third issue, Jonathan indicated that he was often asked whether Billy was still having secretin infusions. The answer was 'no'. After a course of six infusions, they concluded that it was 'a help but not a cure' and stopped, so that Billy could have a full range of diagnostic tests of what his parents believed was his 'dysfunctional immune system'.

Holding therapy and secretin are two examples of a wide range of therapies that have been recommended for autistic children and adopted by desperate parents (National Autistic Society 2003). The interventions that have made a bigger impact have a number of common features. First, treatments often contain an element of rationality: 'holding' may be useful if a child is having a tantrum. Second, even if these approaches do not provide wonder cures for all, they may be of some benefit to some children. Third, the combination of a charismatic scientist or therapist and an evangelical parent helps to gain media attention and wider publicity. Claims of a cure, or of dramatic responses to treatment, are certain to encourage other parents to follow the same approach.

The *post hoc, ergo propter hoc* fallacy is a great friend of alternative treatments. This is the familiar tendency to interpret the fact that one event follows another as indicating that the latter was caused by the former. Parents are liable to confuse association and causation in their assessment of treatments for autism for a number of reasons. First, it is well known that the behaviour of autistic children may fluctuate for no apparent reason. Second, there is a tendency for behaviour to improve over time – particularly in the age range from 6 to 10 (after a more difficult period between 2 and 5) (Wing 1997). Thus, if starting a new treatment coincides with an episodic waning of symptoms, or with a longer-term improvement in the junior school years, the new treatment may be credited for an improvement that would have occurred anyway. Third, it is difficult to isolate the effect of any particular treatment from other factors that may influence behaviour: a child may improve for a range of reasons not connected to the treatment. But when you have invested money, time, energy and, above all, hope, in a particular treatment, it is natural to want to attribute any improvement to that treatment.

In the late 1990s a new trend emerged. Whereas in the past, fairly small groups of parents might take up a particular method, try it and then abandon it, much larger numbers of parents now adopted a more comprehensive alternative outlook, incorporating a range of theories and therapies under the label of 'unorthodox biomedical'. Influenced by the wider climate of distrust in science and medicine, of cynicism about government and of hostility towards corporate power (particularly in pharmaceuticals), a new generation of parents has adopted a high political profile. This is expressed in campaigns – and litigation – against vaccines and vaccine manufacturers, and in the promotion of research along the lines dictated by a new 'unorthodox biomedical' approach.

## The unorthodox biomedical approach

The formation of the Defeat Autism Now! (DAN!) network in Dallas, Texas, in 1995 marked the emergence of a new movement dedicated to challenging the 'biochemical and immunological' causes of autism. The combative name (with obligatory exclamation mark) signalled the militant spirit of the organisers (who include the veteran campaigner Dr Bernard Rimland) and their determination to take on the medical establishment, the government and the corporations in the cause of defeating autism. By 2002 DAN! conferences, held twice-yearly in different American cities, were attracting more than 1,000 attendees, mainly parents, but also professionals and researchers in the field. The DAN! network now links numerous local groups with a similar philosophy from all over the USA and abroad. The support of Dan Burton, Republican senator in Iowa and grandfather of a boy with autism, has provided the movement with an important public platform.

Although there is no umbrella organisation like DAN! in Britain, a number of groups and individuals promote a similar approach. A leading figure is Paul Shattock of the Autism Research Unit at the University of Sunderland; another is Rosemary Kessick, whose organisation Allergy-induced Autism promotes 'gluten-free, casein-free' diets. *The Autism File*, as discussed above, provides detailed accounts of unorthodox biomedical theories and therapies, as well as advertising various clinics and products. The anti-MMR campaign has provided a focus and a source of cohesion for the wider unorthodox biomedical movement in Britain (while MMR is of much less concern in the USA, where parents are more inclined to blame vaccines containing the mercury-based preservative thiomersal for causing their children's problems).

The new parents' movement is a product of the late 1990s. Some of its leading activists have given up careers to devote their often-considerable academic and professional expertise to the cause. The Internet has played a central role in facilitating research and communication: there are now hundreds of websites providing information about the unorthodox biomedical perspective on autism. The new movement is skilled in lobbying and public relations, with good contacts in politics and the media, ensuring a high profile for its campaigns, particularly, but not exclusively, around immunisation issues.

Advocates of the unorthodox biomedical outlook emphasise environmental rather than constitutional factors in the causation of autism, which they believe is a biochemical, metabolic or auto-immune disorder. Indeed some entirely reject the traditional designation of autism as a psychiatric, or even 'neuro-psychiatric', condition, insisting that it is a disorder of the body rather than the mind. Thus, for Jonathan and Polley Tommey, 'autism is a biochemical imbalance, an inflammatory state, a dysfunctional immune system' (Tommey, Tommey, February 2002: 3). Furthermore, it 'is not purely a psychological disorder, a mental illness or a degree of brain damage, but a biological illness'(Tommey, J 2002a: 4). (There are striking parallels with advocacy groups associated with CFS/ME and Gulf War Syndrome, which are similarly insistent on the biomedical origins of the conditions.)

There are a number of curious aspects of the new movement's emphasis on biochemistry and immunology. Although its activists are generally sceptical about medical science and resentful of the medical profession, they put their case in biomedical terms (often of a highly esoteric character) and seek recognition by the medical mainstream. At the same time, they are sympathetic towards a range of 'alternative' health approaches, such as homeopathy and herbalism, and dietary treatments. The result is an eclectic synthesis of biomedical and alternative theories and therapies, with what often appears as a seamless transition from one to the other. While they profess a concern to push medical science forward, their fixation on biochemistry and immunology marks a return to the 1960s and 1970s when significant breakthroughs in these fields put them at the cutting-edge of medical science and raised hopes of even more dramatic therapeutic advances.

For example, in the late 1950s it was discovered that Parkinson's disease resulted from a localised deficiency of the neurotransmitter dopamine. The treatment of patients with encephalitis lethargica with the dopamine precursor L-dopa in the late 1960s was popularised in Oliver Sacks' book *Awakenings* (the film version starred Robert de Niro and Robin Williams) (Sacks 1973). This provoked a wave of optimism that similar neurotransmitter deficits – and similar treatments – might be discovered in other neurological or psychiatric conditions. Similarly, the discovery in 1956 that Hashimoto's thyroiditis resulted from the fact that the patient's body produced antibodies which destroyed its own thyroid tissue prompted hopes that many other diseases whose cause remained obscure might be attributable to the mechanisms of 'auto-immunity'. Unfortunately, these discoveries of neurotransmitters and of auto-immunity, while leading to significant advances in the understanding and treatment of a number of conditions, turned out to be a false dawn for psychiatry (Licinio 2002: 329).

## Biochemical autism

In the golden age of 'metabolic psychiatry' in the 1960s, neurotransmitter theories were advanced to explain schizophrenia and depression (Healy 2002). In this period some researchers suggested that neurotransmitters might be a factor in the causation of autism. Indeed, as the British Medical Research Council's 2001 report observes, 'over the years virtually every neurotransmitter system has been implicated in the pathogenesis of autistic spectrum disorders' (MRC 2001: 41). A number of early studies claimed that urinary levels of serotonin were raised in individuals with autism and suggested that fenfluramine – an early serotonin antagonist (used for a time as a 'slimming pill') – might prove beneficial. Indeed, some studies claimed that it produced improvements in social behaviour and attention span, and reduced motor restlessness. These were not, however, confirmed by further large-scale controlled trials, which also revealed a high incidence of undesirable side effects. Following reports of serious adverse reactions, fenfluramine has now been withdrawn.

In the early 1970s, the dramatic effect of pain-killing drugs such as morphine and heroin ('opiates') was found to be due to the fact that they locked on to specific sites on the surface of brain cells. The discovery of 'opiate receptors' produced a surge of interest in 'endorphins' (naturally occurring opiates or opioids) whose analgesic effect was imitated and enhanced by pain-killing medications. One result was the 'opioid excess' theory of autism, first propounded in the late 1970s by the American neuroscientist Jaak Panksepp, who noticed parallels between the behaviour of experimental animals addicted to opiates and autistic children (Panskepp 1979). Both showed indifference to pain, diminished social interest and extreme persistence in stereotypical behaviours. On the basis of this analogy, he hypothesised that autism might be attributable to an excess of endorphin (or 'opioid') neurotransmitters. In the 1980s studies appeared to confirm higher levels of endorphins in the cerebrospinal fluid of children with autism – particularly those inclined towards self-injurious behaviour (Gillberg, Coleman 2000: 201–2). Trials of naltrexone, an opiate antagonist, claimed improvements both in behaviour and in social interaction. However, further research has failed to confirm any consistent pattern of endorphin levels in autistic subjects, or any consistent benefit from naltrexone (although it may be effective in relieving hyperactivity in some children). (This has not inhibited Dr Panksepp from further speculations: in 1997 he observed that excess opioids produced in response to stress during pregnancy 'appear to lead to some forms of male homosexuality' [Panksepp 1997].)

The 'opioid excess' theory was subsequently taken up by advocates of dietary intervention in autism. In the 1960s the American psychiatrist F.C. Dohan claimed that restricting wheat and dairy products to patients with schizophrenia and children with behavioural disorders resulted in a general improvement. In the early 1980s, the Norwegian biochemist Kalle Reichelt and his colleagues claimed that they had identified abnormal peptides with an opioid effect in the urine of patients with schizophrenia and autism (Reichelt et al 1991). They further claimed that these peptides were the result of the incomplete breakdown of certain proteins in cereal and dairy products: gliadomorphin (from gliaden or gluten in cereal grains) and casomorphin (from casein in milk) (Reichelt et al 1993). They proposed that, in children with autism, bowel inflammation resulting from gluten sensitivity allowed opioid peptides to enter the circulation and produce autistic symptoms, by acting on opiate receptors in the brain. They further postulated that, during pregnancy, circulating opioid peptides derived from the maternal diet could pass across the placenta and, at a critical stage, damage the developing brain of the fetus, producing autism as a result.

In subsequent studies, Dr Reichelt and his team claimed that a gluten- and casein-free diet produced a significant improvement in the behaviour of autistic children (as well as relieving bowel symptoms) (Knivsberg et al 1995). This approach has been popularised in Britain by Paul Shattock and his colleagues in Sunderland, who provide urine testing for opioid peptides with chromatographic techniques, as the basis for dietary intervention (Shattock 1995, Whiteley, Shattock 1997). A number of commercial laboratories in the USA now also offer urine testing, and gluten-free/casein-free diets have become popular with autism parents (Shaw 2002).

In the late 1980s a team of researchers in London analysed the urine specimens of 69 young men (some autistic, some mentally handicapped, some of normal intelligence) and failed to replicate the results claimed by the Norwegians (Le Couteur 1988). More recent studies using more sophisticated techniques have also failed to confirm the finding of exogenous opioid peptides in autistic children (Pavone, Fiumara 1996, Zhang 2000). The opioid excess theory received a decisive blow in April 2003, with the publication of a study by the Edinburgh paediatrician Anne O'Hare and colleagues (Hunter et al 2003). Using a combination of liquid chromatography-ultraviolet-mass spectrometric techniques they failed to detect opioid peptides in either the urine of children with autism or their siblings. The authors suggested that the findings of earlier researchers in this field were unreliable because they used techniques that were neither sensitive nor specific enough to support the conclusions that were drawn from their use.

In 1996 the New York State Department of Health undertook a systematic review of methods of assessment and intervention for young children with autism, and its authoritative report was updated in 1999 (New York State Department of Health 1999). On the question of diet therapies (particularly involving exclusion of milk or wheat products) the authors found only one (of 16 studies) that satisfied their criteria for evidence. Their conclusion was that 'special diets, including elimination diets, are not recommended as a treatment for autism in young children'. The report noted that there were 'no known advantages to special elimination diets for children with autism' and expressed concern that 'they may cause the child to get inadequate nutrition and can be expensive' (New York State Department of Health 1999: Appendix C:14).

These diets may also impose a substantial burden on the whole family. Their advocates insist that they must be followed with military discipline:

> One thing must be made clear right from the beginning of the diet: your child has to stick to the diet rigidly. Evidence has suggested that there tends not to be any middle ground where the strictness of the diet is concerned, it is all or nothing.
>
> (Whiteley, Shattock 1997: 8)

Furthermore, 'compliance needs to be as near to 100 per cent' as possible, for 'at least six months'. The penalty for failure is regression: 'research has shown that children who break the diet do generally tend to regress behaviourally'. However, as discussed above, research has shown that these diets are unlikely to be beneficial for autistic children and, indeed, may be harmful.

From the perspective of mainstream scientific research into autism, the opioid excess theory – a hypothesis based on a weak analogy between rats on heroin and autistic children – never provoked much enthusiasm. However, it subsequently won a new lease of life as the final link in the chain of causality proposed by Dr Wakefield between MMR and autism (see Chapter 9).

### Auto-immune autism?

The quest for an auto-immune mechanism in autism, perhaps linked to an infectious agent, received a boost in the late 1990s with the emergence of the concept of 'Pandas' (paediatric auto-immune neuro-developmental disorder associated with streptococcal infection) (Kurlan 1998). Cases of Tourette's syndrome (characterised by multiple involuntary motor and vocal tics, notably taking the form of obscenities) sometimes occur, or worsen, following throat infections with the bacterium streptococcus. The discovery that some affected individuals had developed antibodies to specific areas of the brain implicated in movement disorders led to the hypothesis that anti-streptococcal antibodies cross-react with brain targets to produce localised neuronal damage, causing the characteristic features of Tourette's. There are some parallels with autism: both conditions have a significant genetic component, and both have in the past been explained in psychogenic terms. A similar mechanism has been suggested to explain the onset of obsessional compulsive disorder in children, in whom it is often associated with tics (it also commonly co-exists with Tourette's) (Murphy, Pichichero 2002). Although the 'Pandas' concept remains controversial, early studies of treatment with intravenous immunoglobulin (IVIG) have been reported as 'promising for the highly selected patient' (Perlmutter et al 1999, Singer 1999). However, it has been recommended that this treatment should be given only as part of controlled double-blind trials and should not yet be considered 'ready for routine use' (Singer 1999: 1138).

Over the past decade there have been a small number of reports claiming to have identified specific auto-antibodies in autistic children, and also claiming dramatic benefits from immunological treatments. Three researchers in the USA – Vijendra Singh, Sudhir Gupta and H. Hugh Fudenberg – have become widely known among parent organisations (all three are referenced in Dr Wakefield's 1998 *Lancet* paper).

Vijendra Singh, associate professor of immunology research at Utah State University, has advanced the hypothesis that a measles virus-induced auto-immune response is a causative factor in autism. In different studies, Professor Singh's team have observed raised levels of antibodies to measles virus and to 'basic myelin protein' – in the lining of nerve fibres – in autistic subjects (Singh et al 1998). In 2002 Professor Singh attracted international attention when he claimed that he had found an unusual MMR antibody in serum samples from 75 autistic children (out of a total of 92 subjects) but no positive results in a control group (Singh et al 2002). Furthermore, 90 per cent of children who were positive for MMR antibodies also had antibodies to basic myelin protein.

Professor Singh's 2002 study was criticised on methodological grounds by Dr Mary Ramsay of the Public Health Laboratory Service (now the Health Protection Agency) in London (DH 2002, Dyer 2002). She considered that the evidence for the specific 'anti-MMR' antibody identified by Singh was 'not credible'. It is also noteworthy that signs of an inflammatory process that generally accompany auto-immune conditions have never been demonstrated in autistic children and that 'demyelination' – the characteristic damage to the myelin sheath surrounding nerve fibres seen in multiple sclerosis – is not a feature of autism. However, on the basis of his contested findings, Professor Singh recommends treating autistic children with a range of immunological treatments, including steroids, intravenous immunoglobulin, plasmapheresis and with sphingomyelin (a product of cattle brains containing myelin) (Singh 1999, 2000). Not surprisingly, in the aftermath of the BSE/CJD outbreak, this treatment has not taken off in Britain.

Sudhir Gupta, head of the immunology department at the University of California at Irvine, has also found a range of immunological deficits in children with autism, for which he recommends treatment with intravenous immunoglobulin (IVIG). In a widely quoted study, he gave ten autistic children IVIG at four-weekly intervals for six months and observed a 'marked improvement in a number of autistic characteristics, including eye contact, calmer behaviour, speech, echolalia, and so forth' (Gupta 1996: 450). In a few children, discontinuation of IVIG resulted in a deterioration, which was reversed when treatment was restarted. The small size of this study, the lack of a control group and the highly subjective character of the assessment of behavioural changes all make it impossible to draw any firm conclusions from this research. Despite this, Professor Gupta provides this treatment for autistic children whose parents flock to see him.

Long retired from his career in clinical immunology, Dr H. Hugh Fudenberg, runs the NeuroImmunoTherapy Research Foundation in Inman, South Carolina. Dr Fudenberg believes that in different individuals autism is the result of immunisations (both measles and rubella), bacterial and fungal gut infections or heavy metal toxins (Fudenberg undated). He further believes that these subgroups can be distinguished by immunological investigations and appropriate therapies thereby instituted. He recommends the use of 'transfer factors', which are said to transfer immunity to autism from a donor to the autistic recipient (Tilton 2000). Transfer factors are 'protein immunomodulators' derived either from cows' colostrum (the fluid expressed before lactation is established after calving) or from human white blood cells (dialysable lymphocyte extract, DLyE), preferably taken from a closely related, non-autistic donor. In a widely quoted paper, he presented the results of treating 22 autistic children with DLyE: 21 showed a significant improvement and 'ten became normal in that they were mainstreamed in school and clinical characteristics were fully normalised' (Fudenberg 1996). With claims like these, it is not surprising that many parents have made their way to South Carolina for this treatment, which is not only very expensive, but carries considerable risks of transmitting blood-borne infections and other adverse reactions.

A number of common themes emerge from a brief survey of the leading promoters of auto-immune theories and immunological treatments for autism. The first is a tendency to make extravagant claims for the explanatory power of auto-immune theories; claims that go far beyond the available evidence. For example, Professor Singh declares that he 'firmly believes' that 'up to 80 per cent (and possibly all) cases of autism are caused by an abnormal immune reaction, commonly known as autoimmunity' (Singh 1999). But scientific theory must be grounded in evidence, not belief, and scientists are obliged to suspend belief until they can substantiate their hypotheses. When Professor Singh suggests that 'a disease is commonly referred to as "autoimmune" when the aetiology and pathogenesis is not well known or established', he implies an 'Alice in Wonderland' approach that allows him to label diseases according to his own hunches (Singh 1999). Professor Singh believes that auto-immune mechanisms explain not only autism, but 'obsessional compulsive disorder, multiple sclerosis, Alzheimer's disease, schizophrenia, major depression, etc' (the 'etc' indicates scope to add further conditions) (Singh 2000). Professor Gupta also takes a broad view of the scope of auto-immune theories: he is also involved in research along similar lines into chronic fatigue syndrome and ageing.

Auto-immunity theorists are inclined to make even more extravagant claims for the scope of their therapies. Professor Singh recommends immunological treatments for all the conditions listed above; Professor Gupta believes that IVIG is the treatment of choice for a range of auto-immune disorders; Dr Fudenberg hails his 'transfer factor' as an effective therapy for attention deficit disorder, HIV/AIDS, chronic fatigue immunodeficiency syndrome, Alzheimer's disease, Gulf War syndrome 'and others'. All three researchers appear to have been ready to jump from preliminary research findings of a highly provisional character to prescribing clinical treatments of unproven efficacy (and uncertain safety) for individuals with autism and other conditions. The contrast with the cautious and circumspect approach of researchers into 'Pandas' is striking.

A third common feature is that these authorities state particularly impressive results in autism. Professor Singh claims that there is 'enormous potential for restoring brain function in autistic children and adults through immunology' (Singh 1999); in Professor Gupta's series of cases, every one was said to have improved on treatment; Dr Fudenberg's claim of a cure rate approaching 50 per cent is the most spectacular of all (Fudenberg 1996). It is a reliable rule of thumb, in the world of health even more than in the marketplace, that if an offer sounds too good to be true, it probably is.

The New York State review was dismissive of these immunologists' claims (New York State Health Department 1999: Appendix C: 11–12). In a 'systematic and thorough review of the scientific literature', the authors found only two articles (those of Gupta and Singh quoted above) that presented information on behavioural and functional outcomes. It found that 'both of these studies had serious methodological flaws and cannot provide acceptable scientific evidence about the efficacy of immune therapies for treating children with autism' (NYSHD 1999: C: 11). It recommended that IVIG and other immunological therapies should not be used for children with autism, emphasising, not only lack of proven efficacy, but that these treatments also posed 'significant health risks' from allergic reactions and transmission of HIV, and hepatitis B and C. The New York report also noted that there was 'no adequate scientific evidence that children with autism have any type of immunologic problems or that they have any immunologic test results that are significantly different than results for the general population' (NYSHD 1999: C:12).

Surveying the history of contradictory and inconclusive immunological findings in patients with autism, in the latest edition of their authoritative text, *The Biology of the Autistic Syndromes*, Christopher Gillberg and Mary Coleman wondered 'whether there will ever be an established immunotherapy for any group of children within the autistic syndrome' (Gillberg, Coleman 2000: 208). In 2001 the British Medical Research Council review noted that 'to date there is not a clear pattern of immunological abnormalities in autistic spectrum disorders, with various abnormalities being reported in a proportion of children'. The review concluded that 'there is no convincing evidence as to a causal relationship between defects of the immune system and autistic spectrum disorders' (MRC 2001: 38).

In some respects the unorthodox biomedical approach reaches even further back into medical history. One preoccupation that is shared by many of its activists is with the toxic effects of the contents of the bowels – a theme that appears in the form of 'autistic enterocolitis' in the works of Dr Wakefield. This phenomenon is now presented in esoteric scientific terms, yet in substance it seems to be little more than a return to the Victorian concept of 'colonic auto-intoxication'.

In the mid-nineteenth century naturopaths in Britain and North America believed that many diseases resulted from toxins absorbed from accumulated faecal matter in the large intestine (Gevitz 1993: 619–20). The ascetic and puritanical health campaigner (and cereal manufacturer) J.H. Kellogg recommended yoghurt to exterminate the harmful bacteria in the colon and roughage (provided by corn-flakes) to expel the toxic waste (Fernandez-Armesto 2001: 51). The famous London surgeon William Arbuthnot Lane went further and undertook surgical removal of the colon (colectomy) to prevent 'intestinal stasis' and 'auto-intoxication' (Porter 1997: 599). He continued performing this drastic operation into the 1930s. Physicians continued to prescribe laxatives in vast quantities to prevent 'intestinal toxaemia' well into the twentieth century (Shorter 1991: 126). Far from looking forward, today's biomedical activists are proposing a return to nineteenth century pseudo-science. This outlook sustains the sort of quackery that flourishes in the form of colonic irrigation – a treatment popularised by the late Princess Diana and still widely available in fashionable clinics and health farms.

## The limitations of parental expertise

At the congressional hearings on autism staged by Dan Burton in April 2000, there was a revolt by parents against what they regarded as the 'patronising propaganda' of the 'mainstream medics'. The following outburst by Karen Seroussi, a promoter of dietary intervention in autism, reveals the anger of the new parents' movement and its intense animosity against what it regards as the medical establishment:

> How dare you patronise us with this kind of information? We are not stupid – we are educated, informed parents who have done thousands of hours of research into autism. We did not come here to be lectured to; we came to be listened to. We are full of ideas that you must hear. We know what happened to our children. How dare you think that you will be able to tell us otherwise.
>
> (Seroussi 2000)

Parents sometimes say 'we know our children better than any doctor or scientist'. I would say that we know our children in a different way. It is a familiar experience with children who are not autistic that they sometimes behave very differently at home and at school; parents and teachers know them differently. With children with autism the problem is more profound. I obviously know my son with autism well; yet in some ways I feel that I do not know him at all – that is the nature of the disorder of autism. He is 11 years old and I have never had a conversation with him and I have very little idea what is going on in his mind, try as I have to work it out. His demeanour is inscrutable and his behaviour is unpredictable. He will sometimes chuckle heartily to himself for no apparent reason, or, more occasionally, will start crying or appear distressed equally inexplicably. He will often react quite differently to what appears to be similar situations and experiences. I fully accept that somebody who has studied the subject intensively and has clinical experience of a large number of people with autism might well know something more about my son than I do.

The experience of having a child with autism qualifies you to speak authoritatively on your experience as a parent of a child with autism: it does not give you any particular insights into the science of autism. Indeed, one of the problems of being the parent of a child with autism is that it gives you little time or energy to study the wider aspects of the subject. In recent years, however, some parents, such as Karen Seroussi for example, have devoted much time to reading scientific papers on autism. But, when such parents demand to be heard – and are heard – in scientific controversies, it is important that the limitations of parental experience and study are recognised.

Modern scientific knowledge in any discipline is complex and highly specialised. The professional understanding of research scientists and clinicians is the product of a long process of study, training and experience. Such knowledge and expertise cannot be acquired through reading papers, downloading information from the Internet and attending occasional conferences, even if parents have 'thousands of hours' in which to pursue these activities (and few have more than a few minutes). At best, parents can acquire what has been called 'narrow-band competence' – familiarity with one small aspect of a subject (Hess 1999: 229). This may allow them to select information that supports a preconceived conviction and presenting this may be effective for campaigning purposes. But a narrow and selective approach can lead to the sort of dogmatic outlook expressed by Karen Seroussi, which is inimical to scientific inquiry and discussion.

In relation to autism research, there are important differences in the perspective of parents and scientists (Schopler 1996). Whereas parents' central concern is with their own children, scientists have to take account of the problems of all children with autism. Parents are interested in practical applications of scientific advances and, watching their children fall ever further behind their peers, they are impatient for short-term results. Researchers are all too aware that, given the limitations of the current state of scientific knowledge of autism, practical applications are likely to be the long-term outcome of advances in the basic understanding of the condition. Parents, whose knowledge about autism is likely to date from the diagnosis of their child, are inclined to jump at novel theories or interventions. Scientists, who base their judgements of new developments and plans for research projects on years of familiarity with the field and on the experience of past studies and experiments, are likely to proceed more cautiously. Scientists are well aware that they may pursue many leads that turn out to be dead-ends before they make some headway. Although parents may justifiably be impatient, they need to be careful they do not short-circuit the scientific process and take their children on journeys that lead to disappointment.

Unfortunately, a number of misunderstandings about the process of scientific research and its presentation have resulted in considerable confusion. There is a wide spectrum of biomedical journals, and these vary widely in quality as well as in content. It is often difficult, even for the experienced reader, to distinguish between a serious journal with a rigorous editorial process and a periodical that is not so discriminating. Inclusion in an internationally recognised electronic database, such as Medline (run by the US Library of Congress), indicates that a journal meets a range of standards and follows an approved process of peer review. Although peer review is no guarantee of quality, and tends to act as a conservative influence, it suggests at least a modicum of quality control. Research published in journals that are not included in Medline is unlikely to make much impact on scientific debate.

The vast majority of studies that are published, even in the more mainstream medical journals, are not directly relevant to clinical practice, either because they are carried out on rats (or other animals) in laboratories, or because they are preliminary studies (Sackett et al 1991: 360). Such researches are designed to clarify a problem rather than provide the solution. The most common outcome of such studies is that they provide information that will be discredited or substantially revised after more advanced testing. In the founding text of 'evidence-based medicine', David Sackett and his colleagues warn that 'one unfortunate consequence of the high concentration of preliminary studies appearing in clinical journals is the premature adoption of innovations' (Sackett et al 1991: 360). This is particularly likely to result from relying on case reports or case series (such as the Horvath paper on secretin or Dr Wakefield's *Lancet* paper). Although such studies may be accurate in announcing the adverse effects of drugs, 'they also introduce what often prove to be useless or harmful treatments, because their methods do not permit discrimination of the valid from the interesting but erroneous'. Thus, the authors conclude, 'they cannot provide, by themselves, a sound basis for clinical action' (Sackett et al 1991: 361).

In the hierarchy of evidence now widely used in medical practice (as follows), 'case reports' occupy the lowest place:

- systematic reviews and meta-analyses;
- randomised controlled trials with definitive results;
- randomised controlled trials with non-definitive results;
- cohort studies;
- cross-sectional studies;
- case reports. (Greenhalgh 2001: 54)

In the world of unorthodox biomedical theories and therapies, there is a preponderance of preliminary and laboratory studies, or clinical studies based on case reports, often published in non-peer reviewed journals. Indeed, some studies are simply launched at conferences of activists and circulated on the Internet, without any process of quality control. Such researches may yield what appear to be impressive results, but parents should be wary of drawing conclusions – and even more wary of implementing treatments – before findings have been validated.

The closer relationship between parents' groups and scientific research into autism may give rise to a number of problems. One is that, under pressure from parents desperate for rapid results, scientists may circumvent the procedures that have been established to ensure adequate standards and to safeguard the public. These procedures require that scientific work is reviewed by peers before publication; that provisional results are confirmed or replicated before claims of significant findings are made; that therapies are subjected to rigorous trials before they are recommended for public consumption. It is unfortunate that for the network of parents promoting the unorthodox biomedical approach to autism, it has become commonplace for all these safeguards to be violated. Scientists who identify with this approach release unpublished data and make claims of unconfirmed findings at public conferences. Parents seize upon provisional reports that appear to confirm some aspect of the unorthodox approach or to validate some therapeutic intervention. There are clear dangers that such prematurely released results are unlikely to be confirmed and that therapies promoted in this way will turn out to be ineffective or to have harmful side effects, or both.

When scientists appeal over the heads of their peers directly to a public lacking in scientific expertise, there is a danger of manipulation. I have attended conferences at which speakers have addressed parents in scientific jargon so dense as to be incomprehensible. Although the object of this exercise appears to be to demonstrate the intellectual authority of the speaker, it means using science to impress rather than to explain, and often leaves parents bewildered and confused. There is also a danger that scientists whose work is not of adequate quality to satisfy the standards of mainstream academic institutions may be able to secure recognition – and increasingly funding – from parents' groups. The danger of abuse is greatest when there are links among scientists, parents' groups and commercial interests, providing diagnostic tests, specialised dietary requirements, food supplements and medications. A common feature of these interventions is that they are inordinately expensive and may constitute a substantial financial burden for some families with autistic children, whose resources are already severely stretched.

Some advocates of the biomedical approach have sought to justify parental experimentation with therapies that have not been fully evaluated. Paul Shattock, for example, notes that, despite professional reluctance to advocate such therapies, parents 'have no such qualms and place themselves at the forefront of experimentation of this type' (Shattock 1995: 1). It would be more accurate to say that they place their children at the forefront of such experimentation. Mr Shattock notes that 'professionals are bound by certain ethical requirements which constrain them from experimentation with such interventions', whereas parents are 'in a desperate situation and will try anything which offers to help their children' (Shattock 1995: 1). But why should children with autism receive a lower standard of protection than others? Children with autism are as entitled as anyone else – indeed, given their vulnerability, more so – to be protected against therapies of unproven efficacy and unproven safety.

On the website of the US-based Autism Biomedical Information Network, Dr Ronald Kallen argues that children with autism should not be subjected to a treatment that is not supported by evidence or which, in the absence of evidence, makes no biological or physiological sense (Kallen 1999, 2000). He further suggests that professionals should not recommend treatments to parents until they have been shown to be beneficial, and without significant side effects, in properly designed trials. Parents are entitled to try any treatment, but they should ask for evidence of both efficacy and safety.

## Full circle

While the unorthodox biomedical movement claims to empower parents, it has done much to restore feelings of parental guilt that had been greatly diminished following the demise of psychogenic theories. While parents were once blamed for their frigid personalities, they now blame themselves for exposing their children to immunisations and other interventions deemed 'toxic' by the new movement. Polly Tommey itemises the offences she believes she committed that caused Billy's autism, in the manner of a penitent confessing sins:

> Billy's problems started off with antibiotics during my pregnancy . . . I did not [breast]feed Billy and he went straight on to formula (cow's milk). He then had the DTP [immunisation against diphtheria, tetanus, pertussis], an insult to his system, then a virus (flu at eight and a half weeks), and then four months of antibiotics (really finishing off the already weak immune system). Then the final trigger – MMR. Billy never recovered from this final insult and autism is the result. I truly believe that the MMR just finished him off. He was probably weakened by all the insults before the MMR but MMR triggered Billy's autism. What on earth were we doing? Deliberately allowing our 13-month-old child with a weak immune system to be subjected to three viruses.
>
> (Tommey, P. 2002: 21)

The guilt expressed by Billy's mother is shared by Jonathan, his father:

> I have deep regret at what we have done to Billy and always say to myself – 'if only I knew then what I know now he would be absolutely fine' – what a waste! But as a caring parent then, with little knowledge of vaccines, I followed the masses.
>
> (Tommey, J. 2002b: 124)

In fact there is no better evidence that Polly and Jonathan Tommey caused Billy's autism through any of these mechanisms than there is for the notion that it resulted from their defective parenting. The fact that the Tommeys have two other children who are not autistic is powerful evidence against both these specious theories. It is iniquitous that the unorthodox biomedical movement should have brought parents in a full circle back to the guilt and self-recriminations suffered by an earlier generation of parents.

# 7

# THE CAMPAIGN AGAINST MMR

If after very careful history-taking ... it can be shown objectively that a child was developing normally and had acquired social and other skills which were within the normal range (and which showed none of the hallmarks of autism) prior to being vaccinated; and if there was no other event which could account for the condition, then *in all probability* the MMR vaccination has played a part in the cause of autism.

(Barr, Limb 1998: 39)

In the aftermath of Dr Wakefield's *Lancet* paper, the campaign against MMR took off as two forces came together under his charismatic leadership. The first was anti-immunisation sentiment. This was a marginal influence in the early 1990s, but it acquired a new momentum and a campaigning focus after Operation Safeguard – the mass immunisation of schoolchildren against measles and rubella in 1994. The second was the growing influence of the unorthodox biomedical outlook among parents, which, as we have seen, included vaccinations as one of the numerous environmental agents believed to contribute to the causation of autism by damaging the immune system. The key figures in this convergence were Richard Barr, the campaigning 'personal injury' solicitor (whose skills in logical argument are illustrated above) who began to take up claims for 'vaccine damages' in the early 1990s and Dr Wakefield himself. Let us look first at Operation Safeguard.

## Operation Safeguard

Operation Safeguard – the immunisation of eight million children between the ages of 5 and 16 in the autumn of 1994 – played an important role in the genesis of the MMR–autism controversy. The campaign (which offered immunisation against only measles and rubella because of a shortage of mumps vaccine) was justified by fears that a generation of schoolchildren was vulnerable to an outbreak of measles (which there was reason to believe might occur in 1995) (Ramsay et al 1994, Salisbury, Horsley 1995). There were also concerns about an increased number of cases of rubella being acquired by pregnant women from young men, who had a low level of immunity to it. Launched in November, Operation Safeguard reached 92 per cent of its target population (CDSC 1995).

There were, however, a number of problems that arose from Operation Safeguard – problems that acquired even greater significance as the wider MMR debacle unfolded. The publicity campaign considered necessary to persuade parents of the need for the MR immunisation inevitably generated popular anxieties. Those promoting the MR could legitimately claim that the public needed to be warned that a measles epidemic was anticipated and warned of the dangers of measles itself. Yet the graphic warnings presented in newspaper and television advertisements, under the banner headline 'Measles Kills', laid the vaccine promoters open to accusations of scaremongering (Roberts 1995). They were accused of exaggerating the seriousness and frequency of complications of measles and of playing down the risks arising from the vaccine itself. As previously discussed, there was already a body of immunisation resisters who could be expected to reject such a health information campaign as tendentious and propagandistic.

While the MR publicity campaign may have convinced many wavering parents in favour of immunisation, it undoubtedly antagonised and further alienated some resisters. The price of the increased awareness of infectious disease and immunisation resulting from Operation Safeguard may have been an increased level of public anxiety about these issues. Formerly a routine matter, issues of immunisation became increasingly problematic for parents, both emotionally and intellectually.

Operation Safeguard also produced a medical maverick, in the form of Dr Richard Nicholson, an ethicist rather than a clinician, and editor of the *Bulletin of Medical Ethics*. In a widely publicised article in his bulletin, Dr Nicholson criticised the mathematical modelling used to predict a measles epidemic in 1995, and argued that this epidemic would not have occurred (Nicholson 1994a, 1994b). In his view, Operation Safeguard was an unjustified and unethical campaign. Dr Nicholson's allegations of conspiracy between the government, the medical establishment and the vaccine manufacturers found a ready resonance among immunisation resisters. Dr Nicholson's article received a comprehensive rebuttal from leading immunisation authorities that insisted that 'given the strong evidence that an epidemic was imminent, it would have been indefensible not to intervene' (Gay, Miller 1995). Yet, for those already inclined towards doubt and suspicion, Dr Nicholson's article provided further encouragement for their nascent anti-immunisation sentiments.

In a review of the MR campaign 12 months after its launch, the Committee on Safety of Medicines (CSM) pronounced a highly favourable verdict. It claimed that the campaign 'successfully prevented an expected epidemic of measles during which it was predicted that there would be around 150,000 cases of measles, 50 with a fatal outcome' (CSM 1995: 10). It noted reports of 1,200 possible adverse reactions, 'most of which were self-limiting' and commented that 'serious suspected reactions were very rare and there were no fatalities'. It concluded that 'the balance of risks and benefits associated with MR vaccine is highly favourable' (CSM 1995: 10). An official survey of the epidemiology of measles published in 1997 presented data showing 'an extremely low incidence of confirmed infections since the national MR campaign in November 1994' and 'a dramatic fall from the incidence before the campaign' (Gay et al 1997: R19). The high level of confidence in MMR was reflected in the decision to launch (in October 1996) a programme for a second dose of MMR in the form of a 'pre-school' booster.

The very success of Operation Safeguard served to disguise the simmering animosities against the immunisation programme, which the campaign itself undoubtedly widened and intensified. It would not be long before these sentiments had a significant impact on MMR uptake.

In the three years following Operation Safeguard a number of different forces came together in the anti-MMR campaign. The first of these was the wider anti-immunisation sentiment that acquired growing cohesion in response to the MR campaign. The formation by Jackie Fletcher of JABS (Justice, Awareness, Basic Support) in early 1994 provided an important link between the earlier anti-immunisation campaigns and the groups that led the later resistance to MMR. Convinced that her son Robert had developed encephalitis, leading to brain damage and epilepsy, after having MMR in 1992, Jackie Fletcher linked up with other parents who believed that their children had been damaged by MMR, or by MR. In the months following Operation Safeguard, JABS compiled a list of several hundred children who had experienced a wide range of adverse reactions, including encephalitis and convulsions, and other neurological deficits.

## Richard Barr: the anti-MMR solicitor

The anti-immunisation campaign was given further impetus by the intervention of lawyers pursuing claims for compensation for damage allegedly caused to children by immunisations. The key figure was the solicitor Richard Barr, who had first come to public attention in the late 1980s for his role in pursuing litigation on behalf of patients who claimed that they had suffered damaging side effects of the anti-inflammatory drug Opren. Although most of these claimants ended up with meagre compensation and the group that Mr Barr encouraged to continue their action ended up with no compensation at all, Mr Barr's reputation as a personal injury lawyer was established (*Guardian*, 1 February 1991). He subsequently took up the causes of alleged victims of the use of organophosphates in farming, ex-soldiers with Gulf War Syndrome, and families who believed that their children had been damaged by immunisations. None of these claimants has yet won any compensation. In the course of the 1990s Richard Barr moved from one firm to another (starting at Dawbarns of Ipswich, then joining Hodge, Jones and Allen of Camden Town and then on to the Manchester-based firm Alexander Harris) always taking his burgeoning portfolio of MMR cases with him.

Mr Barr's first public association with MMR came in 1992 when he represented a 13-year-old boy who developed meningitis after immunisation at boarding school (*Independent*, 16 September 1992). Although this case was dropped, Mr Barr's high profile meant that he soon attracted more claimants, including Jackie Fletcher and other parents who had joined her JABS campaign. By April 1994 he had more than 100 cases and succeeded in winning legal aid for the pursuit of a class action against the vaccine manufacturers, claiming a wide range of adverse effects from MMR, including brain damage, epilepsy, arthritis and immuno-deficiency diseases. In September 1994, the first account of autism attributed to MMR appeared in the British press – 'four children given vaccine from one batch have been diagnosed autistic' (Dyer, *Guardian*, 16 September 1994) – although this story had little immediate impact.

Mr Barr now set about building the case against MMR. According to a sympathetic account, later published in *Private Eye*, 'at last Barr had resources with which to assemble a team to examine the body's complex immune system and how vaccines work' (Mills 2002: 14). This may seem an extraordinary project for a team of solicitors, but the team now included Kirsten Limb, who had a BSc (Hons) and, according to the 'information pack' the team subsequently published, 'an encyclopaedic knowledge of medical matters' (Barr, Limb 1998: 2). 'By 1995', the *Private Eye* account continues, 'the team believed it had found different ways in which the body could be compromised by the simultaneous introduction of three live viruses. They were ready to instruct barristers' (Mills 2002: 14). Only barristers? With this level of scientific expertise, they could have been ready to instruct the Medical Research Council itself.

The 43-page 'information pack' produced by Barr and Limb (Barr, Limb 1998) shortly after the publication of Dr Wakefield's *Lancet* paper undoubtedly attracted many more parents to join the quest for compensation for damage to their children they now attributed to MMR. In promoting the notion of a link between MMR and autism, it can justly claim to be the first manifesto of the anti-MMR campaign – it is still readily available on the Internet. The pack reports the results of a survey of more than 600 parents reporting side effects of MMR and MR vaccines: 'autism is far and away the most common side effect notified to us' (Barr, Limb 1998: 26). Autism was reported by 40 per cent of parents, although only following the combined MMR vaccine. The notion of a link is supported by the observation that 'the word "autism" in relation to its present meaning did not enter the language until about the same time [the 1940s] as wide-scale vaccinations were introduced' (Barr, Limb 1998: 25). Of course, wide-scale smallpox vaccination was introduced in the nineteenth century; wide-scale measles vaccination not until the 1960s; MMR not until the 1980s.

The solicitors' manifesto also promotes the notion of an autism epidemic linked to MMR, which became a central theme of the campaign. 'Is autism on the increase?' the authors inquire, replying that 'anecdotal evidence suggests a huge rise' (Barr, Limb 1998: 27). In the spirit followed by subsequent accounts, they provide numerous anecdotes to support their conviction that there had been a major increase in cases of autism, but no scientific evidence. However, in all the cases reported to these solicitors, autism developed after the introduction of MMR in October 1988.

In another theme that also acquired a wider resonance, the solicitors suggested that the distinctive feature of cases of autism arising from MMR was behavioural regression. Parents reported that their babies appeared to be developing normally until they had the MMR, after which they lost language and other skills and retreated into autism. The solicitors, now apparently experts in autism as well as microbiology, suggest that these cases of 'atypical autism' are likely to be 'a subset', which they estimate at less than 20 per cent of the total (Barr, Limb 1998: 38). (But, to anticipate a continuing problem for the anti-MMR campaign, if MMR was only responsible for a subset, how could it also explain the epidemic?)

When it comes to explaining how various environmental factors, including MMR, might cause autism, the solicitors reveal the influence of unorthodox biomedical views, referring to the auto-immune theories of Singh, Gupta and Fudenberg (see Chapter 6). Although the information pack indicates that the solicitors were 'working with Dr Wakefield' on studies linking measles vaccination to Crohn's disease, it does not suggest inflammatory bowel disease as a possible mediator between MMR and autism.

Given the prominence after February 1998 of the fear that MMR might cause autism, it is worth noting how late this link emerged in the anti-immunisation campaign in Britain. The possibility that vaccines might cause autism was first raised in the USA. Bernard Rimland, the veteran American campaigner, claims that he began to suspect a link between the DPT (diphtheria, pertussis and tetanus) vaccine and autism 'as early as the mid-1960s' (Rimland, 1998). Rimland quotes a book published in 1985, which suggests a link between the recognition of autism as a condition in the USA in the 1940s and the introduction of the pertussis vaccine a few years earlier (the coincidence also noted by Barr and Limb) (Coulter, Fisher 1985). However, US campaigners tend to focus on the risks arising from the use of mercury-containing thiomersal as a preservative in vaccines (which is not included in MMR).

In December 1995 a major feature in the *Sunday Times* magazine provided a publicity boost for the anti-MMR campaign. Yvonne Roberts detailed parents' claims of adverse reactions to the MR vaccine, warning that this could turn out to be 'a catastrophic time-bomb' (Roberts 1995: 17). Illnesses attributed to the MR jab included 'severe epilepsy, arthritis, ME, speech and behavioural problems, inflammatory bowel disease, encephalitis and difficulties with sight and hearing' (Roberts 1995: 17). Although this list does not include autism, the article does discuss the theory of autism as an auto-immune disorder triggered by the measles virus. In a high-lighted box under the headline 'Should your child be vaccinated?' it indicates that risks of measles vaccine 'possibly revealed by new research' include inflammatory bowel disease and a 'possible connection with autism' (Roberts 1995: 20). Research into inflammatory bowel disease provided the unlikely bridge between MMR and autism. The *Sunday Times* feature included a photograph of a youthful Dr 'Andy' Wakefield and provided an extensive account of his claims that Crohn's disease may be caused by measles (Roberts 1995: 20).

Dr Wakefield's presence in the *Sunday Times* feature confirmed that he was already promoting his work in the public realm. Indeed, in October 1994, *The Economist* provided a preliminary account of his forthcoming paper, 'Measles vaccination and inflammatory bowel disease', which was, in an unusual development in academic gastroenterology, launched at a press conference (*The Economist*, 29 October 1994, Wakefield et al 1995, *Guardian*, 28 April 1995). This publicity for Dr Wakefield had two consequences. First, it gave a boost to anti-immunisation campaigns and encouraged popular anxieties about the MMR programme, contributing to the first decline in uptake. Second, it suggested to parents of children with autism and bowel problems that MMR might be the cause of both. Some parents inevitably found their way to Dr Wakefield's clinic: one was Rosemary Kessick, who brought her son William to the Royal Free Hospital in 1996 (Mills 2002: 10).

Already involved with JABS, Mrs Kessick believed that MMR was responsible for both William's bowel problems and his autism, and she received a sympathetic response to this suggestion from Dr Wakefield. This was perhaps not surprising as Dr Wakefield was listening largely to an echo of his own views, with the addition of a link to autism (this was the first case he had encountered). Mrs Kessick was greatly encouraged by seeing Dr Wakefield, and by the improvement in William's behaviour as well as his gastro-intestinal symptoms following Dr Wakefield's treatment (with a diet developed for patients with Crohn's disease). 'Armed with the diagnosis from the Royal Free and feeling vindicated', Mrs Kessick went to see Mr Barr, and William's case joined the growing numbers pursuing compensation. Shortly afterwards Mrs Kessick returned to see Dr Wakefield, not only about William, but with a wider mission in mind: 'She [Rosemary Kessick], Richard Barr and JABS parents then asked Wakefield and his team if they would look at other autistic children who appeared to have identical bowel problems' (Mills 2002: 14). As the *Private Eye* account observes, by late 1996 'the word was out' about a link between MMR and autism (Mills 2002: 14). Before long, the word according to Dr Wakefield was on the lips of parents coming to his clinics, and no doubt influencing the selection of cases in his subsequent study.

The research into the bowel problems of autistic children and the litigation against the vaccine manufacturers brought together the key activists of the anti-MMR campaign: the anti-immunisation campaigner Jackie Fletcher, the parent activist Rosemary Kessick, the lawyer Richard Barr and the gastroenterologist Andrew Wakefield. An article by health correspondent Victoria Macdonald, in the *Daily Telegraph* in November 1996 provided the first public recognition of this convergence (*Daily Telegraph*, 24 November 1996). Under pressure, the Department of Health issued its first circular on this matter, seeking to reassure GPs and other doctors that there was no cause for concern about MMR. It turned out to be the first of many. Thus, by the end of 1996, although the anti-MMR campaign had yet to make a major public impact, its leading figures were all working together, its manifesto had been drafted and it was beginning to get off the ground.

Over the next 12 months or so, the anti-MMR campaign slowly gathered momentum. Mr Barr and Dr Wakefield had written independently to the vaccination authorities at the Department of Health, expressing their concerns about the adverse reactions they believed were resulting from MMR. By the summer of 1997, press and television reports about the alleged MMR–autism links and rumours about Dr Wakefield's impending paper, prompted Tessa Jowell, Junior Health Minister in the newly elected New Labour government, to agree to a meeting. In September, Mr Barr and Dr Wakefield, together with Jackie Fletcher of JABS and Professor John Walker-Smith, senior paediatric gastroenterologist at the Royal Free Hospital, presented their case to the Minister and the Chief Medical Officer, Sir Kenneth Calman, and other officials from the Department of Health. Jowell agreed to establish a forum of independent experts, under the auspices of the Medical Research Council, to evaluate the case against MMR. The first meeting of this committee took place in March 1998, four weeks after Wakefield's *Lancet* paper was published (see Chapter 8).

### The CSM investigation of the solicitors' cases

In response to persistent pressure from Mr Barr, the Committee on Safety of Medicines (CSM) finally agreed to set up an independent working group to investigate the claims against MMR made by Mr Barr's clients (its first meeting took place on 28 February 1998, the day after Wakefield's *Lancet* paper was published). In June 1999, the working party set up to investigate the cases presented by solicitors published its report, based on the evaluation of 92 cases of autism and 15 of Crohn's disease (MCA/CSM 1999a, MCA/CSM 1999b).

The working party's conclusions were based on the solicitors' submissions and the results of questionnaires sent to the children's parents, their GPs and specialists. In evaluating these cases the working party used four key criteria:

- medical confirmation of diagnosis (possible in 81 of the autism cases and 12 of the Crohn's);
- close temporal link between vaccination and onset of symptoms: a cut-off period of six weeks (the time viral replication can be detected after vaccination) was chosen. In 39 of the autism cases and five of the Crohn's, parents reported symptoms within this period;
- the absence of relevant previous medical history (for example, of behavioural abnormality in the autism cases);
- the absence of an alternative cause (such as a family history of the condition in question).

Eight of the 92 autism cases and four of the 15 Crohn's cases fulfilled all four criteria. The working party pointed out that, even in these cases, the apparent link might merely be coincidence. (Given the small number of these cases – a total of 12 – it is unfortunate that the working party did not consider pursuing further clinical investigations of these children. Though problems of selection bias would have limited the scientific value of such a study, it might have gone some way towards countering repeated parental complaints that the authorities refused to pursue clinical studies of the affected children.)

The working party emphasised that the nature of this study made it very difficult to judge whether there was any causal association between the MMR vaccine and the adverse effects that had been attributed to it. It was impossible to compensate for the bias in the selection of cases; there was no (non-immunised) control group with which the frequency and characteristics of the attributed illnesses (autism and inflammatory bowel disease) could be compared. The accounts of the children's illnesses given by doctors and parents often diverged significantly. The working party summed up its conclusion in two sentences, which provoked considerable controversy. First:

> It was impossible to prove or refute the suggested associations between MMR vaccine and autism or inflammatory

bowel disease because of the nature of the information, the self-selection of cases and the lack of comparators.

Second:

Nevertheless, the Working Party found that the information available did not support the suggested causal associations or give cause for concern about the safety of MMR or MR vaccines.

Some commentators considered these statements contradictory (Roberts 1999, Anon 2000). In fact, they are consistent. The first emphasises the limitations of the study and indicates that, on the basis of this information, it was impossible to draw any conclusions about the particular adverse effects attributed to MMR. The second emphasises, in the context of a vaccine that had been given to millions of children in Britain for more than a decade, that what information had been gleaned from these cases gave no cause for concern about its safety.

The key point here is one of continuing importance in the MMR controversy. It is that the onus of proof lies on those alleging that MMR causes specific adverse effects. This is not only because it is impossible to prove a negative: that MMR never causes autism. It is also because we know that MMR, with some 500 million doses given over nearly two decades in numerous countries, has saved thousands of lives and a vast amount of suffering. It would therefore be wrong to suspend the MMR programme, or replace it with an inferior alternative (separate vaccines), without good evidence that it causes the alleged ill effects.

A further study of 900 children whose families were pursuing litigation against the manufacturers of MMR was published in a four-page report in 2001 (Spitzer et al 2001). It was conducted by a team including the Canadian epidemiologist, Walter Spitzer, and the Edinburgh clinical psychologist, Ken Aitken – two late recruits to the anti-MMR campaign. They reviewed the case notes of 493 of these children, of whom 124 were considered ineligible (because the diagnosis of autism was in doubt or because problems preceded MMR). They found that 325 were autistic, although the method of diagnosis was not specified, and that 112 of these had regressed from normal function before MMR to major developmental delay after immunisation.

The key finding of this survey was that the time that elapsed between exposure to MMR and the emergence of autistic symptoms was much longer than in the cases presented in Dr Wakefield's *Lancet* paper. Whereas in the eight cases whose parents attributed the onset of symptoms to MMR in the Wakefield study, the average interval was 6.3 days (range 1–14 days), in the Spitzer cases, the median time from immunisation to the development of symptoms was 1.1 years (range 1 month–7.2 years). (Professor Spitzer excluded cases in which symptoms appeared within 30 days of immunisation, although he found only two of these; a measure that would have ruled out all of the Wakefield's cases!) Professor Spitzer further noted that the median delay from exposure to MMR to diagnosis of autism was 2.5 years. Following this study, supporters of the anti-MMR campaign abandoned the assertion that MMR and developmental regression were 'generally associated in time' – the claim made under the headline 'interpretation' in the summary of Dr Wakefield's *Lancet* paper. Now autism appearing at any time after MMR could be attributed to it. In another article, Professor Spitzer indicated his view that autism could appear 'as late as ten years after immunisation' (Spitzer 2001: 51).

The authors conceded that this brief report was based on an 'obviously unrepresentative and self-selected' sample, although they asserted, unconvincingly, that it was unlikely that this affected their conclusions (Spitzer et al 2001: 163). In its 2001 review of autism research, the Medical Research Council commented acerbically that 'the only conclusions that may be drawn from this study are that MMR is given at 15–18 months of age and the average age at diagnosis of autism in the UK is about four years' (MRC 2001: 30).

Professor Spitzer and Dr Aitken have subsequently emerged as supporters of the anti-MMR campaign: both have been retained as expert witnesses for the plaintiffs in the parents' litigation against the vaccine manufacturers. Although he has formally retired, Professor Spitzer is Emeritus Professor of Epidemiology at McGill University in Montreal, Canada. He has an international reputation for his work on a wide range of issues, including the risks of thrombosis associated with the oral contraceptive pill and the epidemiology of whiplash neck injuries following car accidents. However, he does not appear to have been involved in the study of either immunisation or autism before 1998.

Professor Spitzer has declared that, since meeting 'many of the affected children and their families', he has become 'gradually convinced that the aggregate manifestations of autism are an outcome at least as serious as death' (Spitzer 2001: 54). In his view, 'autistic children act as dead spirits in ostensibly healthy bodies (except for gastro-intestinal complications) *resulting in a very long terminal condition*' (Spitzer 2001: 54, emphasis original). Despite his questionable conviction that autistic children are already dead souls, Professor Spitzer has given his backing to parents who seek compensation from the vaccine manufacturers in the hope that this will give their children a better life.

Dr Aitken, formerly at the Royal Hospital for Sick Children in Edinburgh, now works in private practice as an 'independent consultant child clinical neuropsychologist'. In 1996 he co-authored a textbook on autism, with the Edinburgh psychotherapist and professor of child psychology, Colwyn Trevarthen (Trevarthen et al 1996). In 1998 he was one of the 37 experts invited by the MRC to assess Dr Wakefield's case, and, as it subsequently emerged, the only one to have endorsed it. In 2001, at the request of autism parent activists in Scotland, he was appointed to the expert group set up by the inquiry into MMR conducted on behalf of the Scottish Executive.

In his 'expert group presentation' to the Scottish Executive inquiry and in a 'Q&A' statement published on the Internet, Dr Aitken has indicated his support for the main themes of the anti-MMR campaign (Aitken 2001a, 2001b). These include his belief that the increase in autism is real (rather than a result of improved recognition and wider case definition) and that there has been a particular increase in cases of 'regressive autism'. To support this view he uses the results of a study investigating the potential of the 'checklist for autism in toddlers' (CHAT) as a screening tool for the early identification of autism as though this provides reliable data on rates of diagnosis and regression, which it does not (Baird et al 2000).

Dr Aitken believes that the most likely explanation for the upsurge in 'regressive autism' is some 'new environmental factor', which 'could indeed prove to be MMR vaccines' (Aitken 2001b: 3). Echoing Dr Wakefield's arguments, Dr Aitken considers that there are three 'biologically plausible mechanisms' by which MMR could cause autism: 'an autoimmune reaction'; 'a gastro-intestinal dysfunction'; or 'a direct viral infection of the central nervous system' (Aitken 2001b: 3). His approval of these theories marks a dramatic shift from the view expressed in his 1996 book that 'it now seems certain that the brains of persons who become autistic in their early childhood already had microscopic faults in their development in early intra-uterine life, probably first expressed among cells of the early embryo, in the first month' (Trevarthen et al 1996: 80). This earlier view remains uncontroversial in the world of autism, but is manifestly incompatible with the MMR hypothesis. Dr Aitken has yet to explain how he has come to uphold a fundamental revision in the current understanding of the biology of autism.

In his submission to the Scottish Executive inquiry, Dr Aitken entered into a detailed discussion of issues of vaccine safety and public health (again endorsing the Wakefield line and the demand for separate vaccines) (Aitken 2001a). This was surprising because, as a clinical psychologist, he has no professional expertise in any of the relevant disciplines – paediatrics, microbiology or immunology – (indeed he is not medically qualified).

## The scandal of Legal Aid 'research'

In September 2003, the Legal Services Commission (LSC) called a halt to the MMR case before it went to court because it finally realised it had negligible chance of success. After taking expert advice, the LSC acknowledged that, given the failure of research to establish a link between MMR and autism, the litigation was 'very likely to fail' (LSC 2003). Having already made the 'significant investment' of £15 million in the claimants' unsuccessful attempt to demonstrate this alleged link, the LSC judged that it would be wrong 'to spend a further £10 million of public money' in pursuing the case. The court case that had been planned to start in April 2004 (and had been expected to last six months) was abandoned.

The LSC thus brought to an end a legal campaign that began in 1994, when the former Legal Aid Board agreed to fund a number of claims for compensation for injury allegedly caused by MMR. In its statement on the decision to withdraw Legal Aid, the LSC indicated that the MMR case had been the first in which such funding had been used to finance scientific research. (Apart from the class action over damages claimed to be caused by the benzodiazepine tranquillisers, which also failed, this was the largest single expenditure in the history of Legal Aid funding.) The failure of the research into MMR led the commission to the sober conclusion that 'in retrospect, it was not effective or appropriate for the LSC to fund research'. It emphasised that 'the courts are not the place to prove new medical truths'.

The enormous waste of public funds on the abortive MMR litigation was largely the result of the provision of Legal Aid for 'research' conducted under the direction of a team of scientifically incompetent solicitors.

Following the failure of litigation over the whooping cough vaccine in the 1980s, and the establishment of the vaccine damage payments scheme, there was little interest in pursuing such cases through claims of negligence. Things changed, however, with the introduction into English law of the Consumer Protection Act of 1987, which followed the provisions of the European Product Liability Directive. This meant that manufacturers or suppliers could be held liable for injury caused by their products. Although the new legislation did not require the defendants to prove negligence on the part of the manufacturers, they did have to prove that the product 'caused' or 'materially contributed to' the alleged injury. It was under this legislation that Mr Barr and his colleagues pursued their case against Aventis Pasteur MSD Ltd, SmithKlineBeecham Plc, and Merck & Co Inc, manufacturers respectively of Immravax, Pluserix-MMR and MMR II (three different brands of MMR). (Two of these – Immravax and Pluserix – were withdrawn in 1992 when it was found that the mumps component had caused a number of cases of meningitis.) The anti-MMR campaigners were encouraged by the outcome of the 2001 group action against the blood transfusion authorities over the transmission of Hepatitis C – the first successful case brought under the Consumer Protection Act. All that was required was to prove that MMR 'caused' or 'materially contributed to' autism.

Shortly after Richard Barr joined Alexander Harris in 1999, this firm (and the Nottingham firm Freeth Cartwright) were awarded an 'all works contract' by the LSC, meaning that no other solicitor could take on new MMR cases. As well as handling the bulk of the individual cases, Alexander Harris was responsible for the 'generic' legal case – 'the background research and coordination for the group of cases as a whole' (Alexander Harris 2001). By 2001, Mr Barr was presiding over a 16-strong 'Science and Medical Investigation Team', although closer inspection reveals that these were mostly solicitors or legal executives.

Apart from a couple of former nurses, only three members of the 'Science and Medical Investigation Team' had any scientific qualifications – all at the level of basic university degrees. None had any experience of post-graduate study or research. One of the team, a recent biology graduate, had the specific responsibility of assisting Dr Wakefield's investigations.

Although the full extent of the researches carried out by Mr Barr's team have yet to be disclosed, preliminary court proceedings have revealed the team's activities in a number of areas. Following early hearings, a small number of test cases were selected, with the agreement of both claimants (parents) and defendants (vaccine manufacturers), and these were subjected to a range of investigations. To enable a clinical assessment of alleged bowel inflammation and provide biopsy specimens of the lining of the intestines, the children underwent ileo-colonoscopy under the supervision of Dr Wakefield. They were also required to have lumbar punctures, to provide samples of cerebrospinal fluid (CSF) for further investigation. Because children with autism are unlikely to cooperate with such procedures, they need to be carried out under heavy sedation, if not a general anaesthetic. Parents who were drawn into the legal campaign in the hope of gaining compensation found themselves having to submit their children to distressing investigations.

Given the invasive character of these investigations, and the fact that the procedures themselves carry significant risks, carrying them out for purely litigious purposes raises serious ethical concerns. It is true that, in the course of investigating children with neuro-developmental or gastro-intestinal disorders, specialist paediatricians may sometimes undertake lumbar punctures or colonoscopies. But in these cases the object is to clarify the diagnosis with the possibility that this will lead to some form of beneficial intervention. In other words, investigation is justified by the potential clinical benefit to the child. In the case of the MMR claimants, the indication for investigation was legal not clinical.

It was not surprising that the legal team found that every BUPA hospital in Britain was unwilling on ethical grounds to allow lumbar punctures to be carried out on autistic children in the hope that this might provide some evidence to justify a compensation claim. The anti-MMR lawyers took an extraordinary step to overcome this problem. Ethical considerations notwithstanding, they decided to fly seven children and their parents to Detroit in the USA, where the lumbar punctures were finally done in March 2003. In their submission to the LSC the lawyers claimed that they had acted 'with a determination that can only be admired' (LSC 2003). It seems unlikely that the children with autism, who were dragged half way around the world only to have investigations that turned out to have neither legal nor medical value, shared the lawyers' high opinion of their own actions.

Biopsy, blood, urine and CSF samples taken from the children were subjected to a range of tests – at vast expense – in laboratories retained by the claimants' lawyers. Even when carried out under properly organised scientific conditions, the validity of tests for traces of measles virus – one test widely quoted by anti-MMR campaigners – is highly controversial (see Chapter 8). The tests are not standardised and it is not unusual for them to yield significantly different results in different labs (Afzal 2003); they are also notoriously susceptible to contamination, leading to false positive results. When carried out under the direction of lawyers, by investigators committed to the anti-MMR cause, in the absence of proper 'blinding' and control procedures, they cannot (as the LSC belatedly recognised) be taken seriously. Testing for the presence of 'opioid peptides' – of the sort that Dr Wakefield has hypothesised may mediate between a leaky bowel and autistic behaviour – is also controversial (see Chapter 6). In the end, it appears that the legal team's researches into peptides were stalled because of 'errors in the patenting procedures' of the tests (developed by an anti-MMR campaigner) and could not be included in the preliminary exchange of expert evidence that took place in July 2003.

According to the submissions of the anti-MMR legal team, the results of these investigations were enough to convince their key expert witnesses – Dr Marcel Kinsbourne and Professor John Menkes – to support the case for causation in at least three, and possibly four, of the six children whose investigations had been completed. But who are these expert witnesses?

Dr Kinsbourne is a paediatric neurologist in Los Angeles who testifies frequently in court cases in the USA involving alleged vaccine injury, although he has no record of academic publications in this area. Professor John Menkes is another Californian paediatric neurologist and also a veteran expert witness in cases claiming vaccine injury. In September 2000, Dr Kinsbourne and Professor Menkes joined Dr Wakefield as guests at the second international public conference of the National Vaccine Information Center in Arlington, Virginia (NVIC 2000). The NVIC is a militantly anti-vaccination group, co-founded in 1982 (as Dissatisfied Parents Together; DPT) by Barbara Loe Fisher, who remains its president. The conference brought together anti-vaccination activists, dissident scientists, aggrieved parents and 'personal injury' lawyers from North America and Europe. Other attendees who are also expert witnesses in the anti-MMR case were Paul Shattock, Vijendra Singh and Walter Spitzer. The conference highpoint was the award of special NVIC 'Courage in Science Awards' to Professor Menkes and Dr Wakefield.

Around the time of the appeal against the LSC decision in October, sympathetic journalists acquired details of the anti-MMR legal team's research findings. In an article in the militantly anti-

MMR *Daily Mail*, headlined 'Evidence of MMR risk is "compelling"', Beezy Marsh (a veteran anti-MMR reporter) indicated that, of seven children whose CSF had been tested, three had been positive for measles (one of these was for vaccine strain, the other two indeterminate) (Marsh 2003). She claimed that these 'findings were the closest scientists have come to proving a causal link between the jab, autism and painful gut disorders'. However, rather than indicating the truth recognised by the LSC – that these findings were still a very long way short of proving a causal link – Ms Marsh claimed that 'the authorities were trying to prevent evidence from being made public'.

In an attempt to salvage something from the anti-MMR litigation fiasco, the LSC suggested that it would pass on the fruits of its £15 million investment in the legal team's research programme to the Medical Research Council, which is pursuing research into the causes of autism. It is already clear that this research, which the LSC has decided has no legal value, will also have no scientific value. It is worth recalling that the sum of additional funding granted by the government to the MRC for further research into autism, with a blaze of publicity in February 2002, was £3.5 million.

In a commentary on the MMR litigation some three years before it collapsed, Dr Adrian Rogers, a GP and expert witness, indicated his concern about a case proceeding 'on the hope of finding evidence, rather than on the basis of current information' (Rogers 2000: 5). He considered it extraordinary that public funding should be supporting these cases on the basis of research that had not even taken place, particularly when the proposed 'link was so thin as to be theoretical'. As he suggested, on this basis, all sorts of groups could seek funding for research in the hope that his might provide the 'legal basis for a putative claim'. He concluded that 'causation, if it is to be legally proven, requires more than sympathy and public funding' and proposed that 'compensation should wait until causation, if it can be established, has been established properly' (Rogers 2000: 6). Unfortunately, despite these warnings, the anti-MMR campaign, which had come to provide a substantial income for numerous lawyers, scientific researchers and expert witnesses, carried on for a further three years.

By late 2003, while campaigners vowed to continue the quest for compensation, it was clear that, despite spending £15 million over nearly a decade, the combined efforts of Mr Barr, Dr Wakefield and all the highly-paid experts had failed to establish a causal link between MMR and autism in a single child.

# 8

# THE *LANCET* PATER

We identified associated gastrointestinal disease and developmental regression in a group of previously normal children, which was generally associated in time with possible environmental triggers.

(Wakefield et al 1998: 637)

We did not prove a link between MMR vaccine and this syndrome ['autistic enterocolitis'].

(Wakefield et al 1998: 641)

Dr Wakefield's landmark paper, published in *The Lancet* on 28 February 1998, provided the missing link in the theory that MMR was responsible for the supposed 'autism epidemic'. That link was 'autistic enterocolitis' – a novel and distinctive form of inflammatory bowel disease found in children with autism and other developmental disorders. Dr Wakefield was the 'senior scientific investigator' in the Royal Free research team and the paper's lead author. A dozen co-authors included paediatric gastroenterologists Simon Murch and Mike Thomson, who did the colonoscopies, child psychiatrist Mark Berelowitz, and Professor John Walker-Smith, who was the 'senior clinical investigator'. Dr Wakefield and his colleagues believed they had made a discovery of historic significance; it was rumoured that some of them wondered aloud whether they might win a Nobel Prize or some similar recognition if their bold hypothesis was vindicated.

The paper was based on the investigation of 12 children, who were said to have been consecutively referred to Dr Wakefield's clinic at the Royal Free Hospital with a history of diarrhoea, abdominal pain, bloating, and food intolerance. The dozen included only one girl; in ten cases the diagnosis was autism or 'autistic spectrum disorder'; in two there was a suspicion of 'post-viral encephalitis'; and in one the diagnosis was uncertain between autism and 'disintegrative disorder'. Examination of the lining of the large and small intestine through a fibre-optic endoscope (ileo-colonoscopy) passed up the rectum (under sedation) revealed a distinctive pattern of inflammation (non-specific colitis) associated with enlarged lymph glands at the end of the small intestine (ileal lymphoid nodular hyperplasia). Microscopic examination of biopsy specimens confirmed chronic inflammatory changes. Furthermore, the authors reported that the parents of eight of the children believed that their behavioural symptoms, characterised as 'regression', began shortly after the MMR immunisation (on average after 6.3 days). They suggested that, in these children, the measles virus (present in an attenuated form in the MMR vaccine) might have produced bowel inflammation, allowing toxic peptides to 'leak' into the bloodstream and hence pass to the brain, causing autism.

The authors conceded that they had not proved a link between MMR and 'autistic enterocolitis'. However, they considered that the chronic inflammatory features they had identified in both the small and large bowels of these children 'may be' related to neuropsychiatric dysfunction. The interpretation offered in the summary at the head of the report, as quoted above, was that the authors had 'identified associated gastro-intestinal disease and developmental regression in a group of previously normal children, which was generally associated in time with possible environmental triggers' (Wakefield et al 1998: 637). The only 'environmental trigger' identified in the report was MMR immunisation, which was linked by eight of the children's parents to the onset of their disturbed behaviour.

## An acrimonious debate

There were two unusual aspects to the publication of the Wakefield paper and both contributed to the subsequent furore. The first was that it was accompanied by a critical commentary by Robert Chen and Frank DeStefano, two American vaccine specialists (Chen, DeStefano 1998). The second was that it was launched at press conference at the Royal Free Hospital. Let us look at these in turn.

As Richard Horton, editor of *The Lancet*, has indicated in his reflection on the 'acrimonious debate' that erupted following his decision to publish the Wakefield paper, he was well aware of its controversial character (Horton 2003: 207). The substance of Dr Wakefield's MMR–autism thesis had already been widely leaked and

*The Lancet's* peer reviewers had raised concerns about the study's methods and interpretations, as well as about the dangers of undermining public confidence in immunisations. Dr Horton insisted that the paper was revised to clarify that its authors had no proof that MMR caused autism, following which it was published under the label of 'early report' to 'highlight its preliminary nature' (Horton 2003: 208). Furthermore, he commissioned two US vaccine experts, Robert Chen and Frank DeStefano to write 'Vaccine adverse events: causal or coincidental?' – a brief but devastating critique of the Wakefield paper published in the same issue of *The Lancet* (Chen, De Stefano 1998).

Chen and DeStefano first indicated the excellent safety record of MMR in hundreds of millions of people worldwide over three decades. They questioned whether the newly identified syndrome of autistic enterocolitis could be considered clinically distinctive: 'no clear case-definition was presented, a necessary requirement of a true new clinical syndrome and an essential step for future research' (Chen, DeStefano 1998: 612). They emphasised that the authors had not confirmed the presence of vaccine virus in the tissues of their patients. They suggested that 'selection bias' might have resulted from the referral of children to the clinic of 'a group known to be specially interested in studying the relation of MMR vaccine with inflammatory bowel disease' (Chen, DeStefano 1998: 612). They noted that it is usually difficult to date precisely the onset of a syndrome such as autism, and wondered whether 'recall bias' may have resulted from parents attempting to relate the onset of their child's problems to an unusual event such as a coincidental vaccine reaction. They also pointed out that, although Dr Wakefield and his colleagues postulated that MMR might lead to inflammatory bowel disease, which, in turn, might cause autism, in almost all the cases reported in their paper behavioural changes preceded bowel symptoms. The time course of these pathological processes was also curious: in one case the effect of MMR on behaviour was evident within 24 hours – faster than any known process of infection-induced vasculitis (the underlying pathology postulated as the cause of 'autistic enterocolitis, a type of process that unfolds over several weeks).

In conclusion, Chen and DeStefano warned presciently that, if claims of adverse events resulting from vaccines were not properly substantiated, there was a danger that vaccine-safety concerns may 'snowball into societal tragedies when the media and the public confuse association with causality and shun immunisation' (Chen,

DeStefano 1998: 612). Many of these themes were taken up and expanded in subsequent letters to *The Lancet*.

In retrospect, Dr Horton conceded that the publication of Dr Wakefield's paper in *The Lancet* gave it 'more credibility than it deserved as evidence of a link between the MMR vaccine and the new syndrome' (Horton 2003: 209). Yet, while he defended his decision to publish the paper, he unreservedly admitted to 'a failure to manage the media reaction' – a failure that started with the now notorious Royal Free press conference.

The press conference was an extraordinary event. Journalists were treated to a special introductory video prepared by the Royal Free press office and the Dean of the Medical School, Professor Arie Zuckerman, himself a vaccine specialist, presided over the conference. (Professor Walker-Smith refused to attend, indicating that he disapproved of medical research being debated prematurely in the mass media. He has recalled that the only enthusiasm for the conference came from Dr Wakefield and his staunch ally Professor Roy Pounder, senior adult gastroenterologist at the hospital [Walker-Smith 2003: 241].)

Dr Wakefield seized the next day's headlines with his sensational recommendation that parents should reject the MMR immunisation and give their children each of the three components separately, 12 months apart (*The Times*, 27 February 1998, *Daily Telegraph*, 27 February 1998). This recommendation was not included in the *Lancet* paper and is in no way supported by it. Such a programme of vaccination has not been introduced anywhere in the world and there is no evidence to justify any particular interval between vaccinations. It was immediately repudiated by Professor Zuckerman and by the paediatricians in the Wakefield team. Dr Simon Murch, Dr Mike Thomson and Professor Walker-Smith subsequently wrote to *The Lancet* to disassociate themselves from Dr Wakefield's call for separate vaccines (Murch et al 1998). Not a single member of the team publicly endorsed Dr Wakefield's anti-MMR stand. Yet, as the press conference broke up in rancour, the campaign against MMR received its biggest boost so far.

Five years later Richard Horton was still smarting from the 'vituperative attack and personal rebuke' he experienced as a result of his decision to publish the Wakefield paper (Horton 2003: 213). Many critics complained that *The Lancet*'s process of peer review should have exposed the weaknesses of the paper and prevented its publication. Dr Horton insists that the role of peer review is not to judge the validity of a piece of research – that can only be verified by other scientists – but to comment on the importance of the issue under investigation and on the design and execution of the study (Horton 2003: 213). He decided to publish Wakefield's paper, not because he believed it to be true, but because it raised an important question that required urgent verification. Dr Horton has argued the important principle that medical journals must uphold free expression in scientific debate even if this creates problems for public health. He maintains that to have refused to publish Wakefield would have been an act of censorship. But, as Chen and DeStefano and many others have pointed out, there were basic errors in design, execution, analysis and interpretation in the Wakefield paper. Dr Horton indicates elsewhere that, every year, *The Lancet* publishes 500 out of 10,000 papers that are submitted: this is not censorship but editorial judgement (Horton 2003: 307). Indeed, when Dr Wakefield submitted his follow-up paper, including a further 48 cases, Dr Horton exercised this discretion and rejected it (it was finally published in the *American Journal of Gastroenterology*; Wakefield et al 2000).

## MMR and the Medical Research Council

Although the Royal Free press conference projected the MMR–autism debate onto the national stage, and Dr Wakefield gained a growing status among anti-immunisation campaigners and parents of autistic children, he made little headway in convincing his medical and scientific colleagues of his case. In March 1998, at the request of Sir Kenneth Calman, Chief Medical Officer, the Medical Research Council (MRC) convened an ad hoc group of 37 experts, drawn from the spheres of virology, gastroenterology, epidemiology, immunology, paediatrics and child psychiatry, to review the associations suggested by the Royal Free team between measles virus and MMR on the one hand, and between inflammatory bowel disease and autism on the other (MRC 1998). The group's meeting was chaired by the pathologist Professor Sir John Pattison (a veteran of the mad cow crisis); Dr Wakefield and epidemiologist Scott Montgomery (one of the Royal Free team) attended the meeting to present and discuss their case.

The group first considered the laboratory evidence produced by the Royal Free group for the hypothesis that measles virus caused inflammatory bowel disease and noted that 'the most sensitive molecular genetic techniques were negative in the hands of all groups' (see Chapter 9) (MRC 1998: 2). They emphasised that further studies 'must involve independent laboratories testing the same specimens, using full controls and a range of techniques with agreed experimental protocols' (MRC 1998: 2). When considering the epidemiological evidence claimed to link viral infections and inflammatory bowel disease, the group found no correlation between measles or mumps infection alone and Crohn's disease and ulcerative colitis. The experts agreed that there was some correlation between the occurrence of measles and mumps infection within the same year and the later incidence of inflammatory bowel disease. However, they considered existing studies limited and recommended further examination by independent groups.

On autism, the group considered the *Lancet* paper and emphasised the point that autism commonly becomes apparent in the second year of life – at around the time children receive MMR. However, the group insisted, 'such coincidence does not imply a causal link'. They pointed out that, whatever the trends in the incidence of autism, they bore no relationship to the introduction of MMR. They considered that the proposed 'leaky bowel'/opioid excess mechanism was 'biologically implausible' (MRC 1998: 3). They further pointed out that the supposedly distinctive pattern of 'lymphoid nodular hyperplasia' identified by the Royal Free group was a common and benign condition in children. Finally, it was argued that the findings of abnormally low levels of some immunoglobulins (IgA) in four out of the twelve children was a simple error resulting from the use of adult normal ranges (when using appropriate paediatric ranges, only one child had a low IgA level) (Richmond, Goldblatt 1998).

After a day-long meeting the experts concluded that there was no current evidence linking MMR and autism. They thought that 'it would be surprising if the link had not been noted in other countries with good diagnostic facilities for autism where MMR has been widely given for many years' and suggested that 'further research on an international basis would settle this matter' (MRC 1998: 3). The expert group advised the Chief Medical Officer that there was no reason for a change in current MMR vaccination policy, as had been recommended by Dr Wakefield. However, they proposed more research on both inflammatory bowel disease and autism. These conclusions were sent in summary form to every doctor in the country in a letter from the Chief Medical Officer on 27 March (Calman 1998).

Dr Wakefield later complained that he felt he had been 'set up' at this meeting (Mills 2002: 17). He claimed that the 37 experts had all been 'picked by the government' and that he and Dr Montgomery had had to face them 'alone'. He felt that a nine-hour meeting fell short of the detailed scrutiny he had hoped for.

Following the March 1998 meeting, the MRC set up an expert subgroup to steer and monitor research in inflammatory bowel disease and autism. This subgroup included leading figures in the relevant disciplines and it invited other specialists to attend particular meetings: these included Dr Wakefield, and his co-authors Professor John Walker-Smith and Dr Simon Murch. In its report in April 2000, the subgroup noted further evidence from the Royal Free group of 'a classic pan-colitis associated with severe constipation and immune dysregulation in a group of children with developmental disorders' (MRC 2000, Wakefield et al 2000).

This study compared a series of 60 'consecutive' cases of 'autistic enterocolitis' (including the orginal 12), with a control group of 37 developmentally normal children undergoing ileo-colonscopy. Given the controversy still raging around the *Lancet* paper, it was curious that the new study included no information about MMR or any other immunisation history. The study confirmed 'an endoscopically and histologically consistent pattern of ileo-colonic pathology' in 'a cohort of children with developmental disorders' (Wakefield et al 2000: 2294). It also recorded results of investigations suggesting minor immunological abnormalities. The authors described a subtle 'new variant' inflammatory bowel disease, lacking the specific features of either Crohn's disease or ulcerative colitis. They again drew attention to the association of this pattern of bowel disease with 'a developmental disorder that was associated with a clear history of regression' – a loss of skills after a year or more of normal development. They concluded that 'this syndrome [autistic enterocolitis] may reflect a subset of children with developmental disorders with distinct etiological and clinical features' (Wakefield et al 2000: 2294).

This study was open to the same charges of selection bias as the *Lancet* paper. It was also criticised on the grounds that the control group was not properly matched for age. Apart from providing a fuller picture of the supposed new syndrome of 'autistic enterocolitis', it added little to the continuing MMR–autism controversy. The MRC report concluded that 'the case for "autistic enterocolitis" had not been proven' (MRC 2000: 4). It commented that the Royal Free studies had been performed in a 'self-selected group of patients and the histological finding of ileal lymphoid-nodular hyperplasia may have been secondary to severe constipation' (MRC 2000: 4).

The subgroup concluded that, in the 18-month period following Dr Wakefield's *Lancet* paper, 'there had been no new evidence to suggest a causal link between MMR and inflammatory bowel disease/autism' (MRC 2000: 5). It conceded that much remained unknown about these conditions and that MRC support for research in these areas, particularly inflammatory bowel disease, was weak. It made a series of specific recommendations for future research.

## Testing the MMR–autism hypothesis

In the concluding 'discussion' section of their *Lancet* paper, Dr Wakefield and colleagues suggested that further investigations were needed to examine the syndrome of 'autistic enterocolitis' and 'its possible relation' to MMR (Wakefield et 1998: 641). They indicated two directions for further research. First, the authors observed that if there were a causal link between MMR vaccine and this syndrome 'a rising incidence might be anticipated after the introduction of this vaccine in the UK in 1988'. They considered that published evidence was inadequate to answer this question, inviting further epidemiological research to clarify it. Second, they reported that 'virological studies' (presumably those later reported by the team headed by Professor John O'Leary in Dublin, Ireland) were 'underway'. Let us now examine the outcome of attempts to substantiate the MMR–autism hypothesis through researches in these areas.

In its responsibility for vaccine safety, the Medicines Control Agency commissioned an epidemiological study to investigate the question of whether there was an increase in cases of autism in Britain following the introduction of MMR. Dr Wakefield's challenge to analyse any rise in incidence was taken up by Professor Brent Taylor, community paediatrician at the Royal Free Hospital, and a team including vaccine specialist Dr Elizabeth Miller and Open University statistician Dr Paddy Farrington. Their results were published in *The Lancet* in June 1999 (Taylor et al 1999a).

They identified all known children with an autistic spectrum disorder born between 1979 and 1998 in eight North Thames health districts – 498 children in all – and studied their medical and vaccination records. They found that:

- although the number of cases of autism had increased steadily since 1979, there was no sudden 'step-up' or change in the trend line after the introduction of MMR in 1988;
- there was no difference in age at diagnosis between the cases vaccinated before 18 months of age, after 18 months of age, and those never vaccinated;

• there was no clustering of developmental regression in the months after vaccination.

They concluded that 'our analyses do not support a causal association between MMR vaccine and autism' (Taylor et al 1999a: 2026). The authors themselves acknowledged two limitations of their study. They could not verify the diagnoses of autism in all cases and they may have missed some cases. They relied on clinical notes of variable quality and many did not contain systematic or regularly updated information, which would have allowed independent validation of diagnosis. Despite making 'substantial efforts' to identify all cases, they may have missed some children who were not known to local health or education authorities. However, it is unlikely that these factors significantly affected the overall results.

In a letter to *The Lancet*, Dr Wakefield criticised the Taylor study on three grounds (Wakefield 1999). He claimed that the statistical methodology used ('case-series') was inappropriate to detect temporal associations between vaccination and conditions, such as autism, characterised by an insidious onset and delay in diagnosis. On the contrary, the authors replied, this method was particularly suitable for this sort of study, which has a good record of revealing rare adverse effects (Taylor et al 1999b). Dr Wakefield's second objection focused on the authors' judgement that one finding – that of a marginally significant raised incidence of parental concern between 0 and 5 months after MMR – was a statistical artefact. The authors claimed that one such finding (out of 14) might have been expected by chance, and that it could be explained by 'the combined effect of approximate recording of parental concern at 18 months and a peak in MMR vaccinations at 13 months'. Finally, Dr Wakefield made the accusation that the authors had 'failed to declare' the fact that some of the children in the study may have received MMR as a result of a catch-up campaign. The authors' rebuttal was that these children had been identified and that in all cases in which the age of first parental concern was recorded, it preceded vaccination.

If epidemiological studies failed to support the MMR–autism hypothesis, what about the virological studies? During 2002 two papers based on studies of intestinal biopsies on Dr Wakefield's 'autistic enterocolitis' patients by a team lead by Professor John O'Leary in Dublin were published.

In the first paper, published in February, the researchers claimed to have identified fragments of the measles virus in intestinal tissues of 75 out of 91 children with inflammatory bowel disease and developmental disorder (Uhlmann et al 2002). However, this study did not indicate whether the children had had measles or MMR. The authors did not indicate whether they had found whole measles virus, whether of wild or vaccine strain, or any other viruses, such as mumps and rubella. Many commentators wondered whether inadvertent sample contamination or some other technical error with the notoriously difficult reverse transcriptase polymerase chain reaction assays might explain these results (Afzal et al 2003). The study was also criticised on the grounds that the controls were not matched for age or time since vaccination. Others observed that, even if these findings were confirmed and replicated, the presence of measles virus fragments in the gut would not prove that they caused either inflammatory bowel disease or autism.

In response to the controversy generated by his paper, Professor O'Leary issued a statement insisting that he had 'not set out to investigate the role of MMR in the development of either bowel disease or developmental disorder, and no conclusions about such a role could, or should be, drawn from our findings' (O'Leary 2002a).

In a presentation in June 2002 to a US congressional committee Dr Wakefield claimed that a new study, due to be published by Professor O'Leary, had confirmed that the measles virus present 'in the diseased intestinal tissues of children with regressive autism' was indeed derived from the MMR vaccine (Wakefield 2002a). For Dr Wakefield, these studies constituted 'a key piece of evidence in the examination of the relationship between MMR vaccine and regressive autism'. Professor O'Leary, however, promptly rejected Dr Wakefield's interpretation of his work, insisting that it 'in no way establishes any link between the MMR vaccine and autism'. (O'Leary 2002b). Indeed, he strongly recommended that parents should give their children MMR[1].

An abstract (summary) of the new O'Leary study was duly presented at the annual meeting of the Pathological Society of Great Britain and Ireland in Dublin in July 2002. This was a pilot study designed to discover whether the measles virus RNA found in the

---

1 It is interesting to note that Professor O'Leary's repudiation of the claims, made on his behalf by Dr Wakefield and his supporters, has never been acknowledged by the anti-MMR campaigners, who continue to cite O'Leary's research in support of the MMR–autism thesis, in explicit defiance of his statements to the contrary.

guts of children in the earlier study originated in wild measles or from immunisation. The paper described a technique for discriminating between two closely related genome sequences, which the authors claimed could distinguish between wild and vaccine strain measles (by identifying a single nucleotide at position 7901 of the genetic code of the wild measles virus). They found vaccine-strain measles virus in the gut biopsies of 12 children with inflammatory bowel disease and development disorder (and confirmed wild measles strain in brain specimens of three patients with SSPE – a rare complication of measles). They concluded that 'this pilot study corroborates our earlier findings of an association between the presence of measles virus and gut abnormalities in children with developmental disorder, and indicates the origins of the virus to be vaccine strain' (Shiels et al 2002).

However, an immediate response to this study from the WHO collaborating centre for measles in the UK challenged the validity of the technique used by O'Leary's team. This indicated that the method used was not able to distinguish between wild and vaccine strains (it could result in several wild strains being incorrectly classified as vaccine strains). 'Consequently', it concluded, 'the technique described does not reliably discriminate between wild and vaccine measles virus' (Brown et al 2002). When presented with this information at the US congressional hearings on autism, Dr Wakefield accepted that if this method could not reliably make distinguish the two different forms of measles, then the conclusion drawn by the paper was not justified. The first piece of evidence promising some support to the hypothesis advanced by Dr Wakefield in 1998 was thus discredited even before publication.

## MMR safety

In January 2001 Dr Wakefield adopted a radically different tack in the campaign against MMR. He now turned to the field of public health and vaccination policy, questioning whether appropriate safety procedures had been followed when MMR was introduced into Britain in the late 1980s. In a paper written with his Royal Free colleague, epidemiologist Scott Montgomery, Dr Wakefield claimed that the trials carried out on MMR before it was licensed in Britain involved monitoring children for side effects for only 28 days (Wakefield, Montgomery 2000). They also claimed that the authorities had not taken account of the problems of 'viral interference' arising from using the combined MMR vaccine and that early studies had missed or ignored evidence of gastro-intestinal side effects of MMR.

Entitled 'MMR vaccine: through a glass, darkly'[2] the Wakefield and Montgomery paper provoked a storm of controversy.

It was published in the *Adverse Drug Reactions and Toxicological Reviews*, a highly specialist (and now defunct) journal with a regular readership estimated at around 300. The editors of this journal, anticipating a critical response to the article, published it together with the comments of four reviewers. (Critics subsequently pointed out that, although the reviewers were distinguished in their own fields, they did not include a vaccine specialist.) The most significant comment came from Dr Peter Fletcher, a former head of the Committee on Safety of Medicines, who substantially endorsed the case made by Wakefield and Montgomery and concluded with the damning judgement that 'the granting of a produce licence [for MMR] was premature' (Fletcher 2001: 289). In the subsequent discussion, another supporter of the anti-MMR campaign emerged: Dr Stephen Dealler, consultant microbiologist at Burnley General Hospital in Lancashire (Dealler 2001). A veteran of the BSE/CJD controversy, in which he emerged as a protégé of Professor Richard Lacey (whose maverick reputation appeared to be enhanced when the nightmare scenario he had long predicted came, at least in part, to pass), Dr Dealler had now become a supporter of Dr Wakefield's theory of autism (see Fitzpatrick 1998: 45–8). He had already published a comprehensive endorsement of unorthodox biomedical approaches to autism on the Internet (Dealler 1999).

Recognising that his most recent paper might not otherwise attract public attention, Dr Wakefield launched the article at a press conference and released copies of the paper to the mainstream media before either public health authorities or doctors involved in giving vaccinations had a chance to read it. Another stormy press conference guaranteed a blaze of publicity (Abbasi 2001).

The Wakefield/Montgomery paper prompted forceful rebuttals from vaccine authorities. On behalf of the Medicines Control Agency, Arlett and Bryan insisted that the MMR trials had followed up children for between six and nine weeks (and, in some studies, for longer) (Arlett, Bryan 2001). They accused Wakefield and

---

2   The title is derived from the epistles of St Paul: 'For now we see through a glass, darkly; but then face to face: now I know in part; but then shall I know even as I am known' (Corinthians I; 13:12).

Montgomery of errors of statistics and interpretation of key surveys, and claimed that they had missed or ignored other important studies. A scathing review from the Public Health Laboratory Service (now the Health Protection Agency) concluded that 'overall, we find this paper lacking in a coherent scientific rationale, selective in the reporting and interpretation of other work and statistically invalid' (Miller, Andrews 2001). Paediatric vaccine specialists dismissed the concerns raised by Wakefield and Montgomery as 'idiosyncratic' and questioned the authors' tactics in presenting their paper to the popular press before most clinicians had a chance to read it in a peer-reviewed journal (Elliman, Bedford, 2001).

Two distinct issues were confused in the discussion of 'interference' (Arlett, Bryan 2001, Wakefield, Montgomery 2001). One is the question of whether there is a higher incidence of adverse reactions with the combined vaccine, compared with vaccines given separately. Contrary to Dr Wakefield's claims, the consensus emerging from a number of studies is that there is not (Halsey 2001). For the MCA, Arlett and Bryan insisted that there was no convincing evidence of either chronic gastro-intestinal problems or autism resulting from MMR (Arlett, Bryan 2001). The second is the question of 'immunological interference': does giving three antigens together lead to a diminished antibody response to each one? According to the review by the American Academy of Pediatrics, 'although early studies showed the potential for some interference between these vaccine viruses as indicated by reduction in the mean antibody response to one or more of the components in the combined vaccines, adjusting the titres of the vaccine viruses resulted in similar responses for the combined and separate administration of these vaccines' (Halsey 2001: 25). Arlett and Bryan pointed out that, in 30 studies of the combined MMR vaccine before its introduction in Britain, no problems of interference had been identified. Furthermore, the effectiveness of post-licensing surveillance had been confirmed by its success in identifying, as a rare adverse reaction, ITP (idiopathic thrombocytopenic purpura – a rash associated with a blood abnormality, which usually resolves spontaneously) at a rate of one in 24,000 cases (Miller 2001).

In the subsequent discussion about the safety of MMR a number of issues arose (although none shed much light on the MMR–autism hypothesis). One set of concerns – promoted at first by the wider anti-immunisation movement – focused on the withdrawal in Britain in 1992 of two brands of MMR that used a mumps component derived from the Urabe strain of the virus. In 1988, before the introduction of MMR in Britain, a study in Canada and the UK reported the occurrence of aseptic meningitis following immunisation with the Urabe strain mumps vaccine, at a rate of between one in 100,000 to one in 250,000. Given that this rate of meningitis was much lower than that occurring with natural mumps (which MMR had been shown to prevent) it was preferable to proceed with the introduction of MMR. Furthermore, it was not, at that time, clear that any alternative vaccine was safer. However, although passive surveillance procedures showed a very low risk, a more intensive study in 1992 in the Nottingham area revealed a higher incidence of aseptic meningitis – at a rate of one in 3,000 – following MMR (Miller et al 1993). Accordingly, the vaccine authorities decided to switch to using only brands of MMR containing the Jeryl Lynn strain of mumps (which had not been linked to cases of meningitis). In response to continuing claims of government perfidy in introducing MMR including Urabe (on the grounds that it was known to cause aseptic meningitis in rare cases), it has been pointed out that, if Jeryl Lynn had not been available, it would still have been preferable to carry on with MMR include Urabe as the benefit from reducing the risk of mumps far exceeded the risk of vaccine-related meningitis.

Another controversy arose from official attempts to promote studies of MMR safety in general as evidence against claims that it caused autism. The most popular study in this regard comes from Finland – a country that introduced a two-dose MMR programme in 1982 and now claims to have virtually eradicated these three diseases. Long-term population-based passive surveillance studies found that no cases of developmental regression had been reported as resulting from MMR in 1.8 million children (Peltola et al 1998, Patja et al 2000). It is true, however, that because people in Finland had no reason to suspect that MMR might be associated with autism, they would be unlikely to report it as an adverse reaction. Dr Fletcher, among many others, was critical of the government's use of such 'negative studies as absolute evidence of safety'. Nevertheless, the large-scale, long-term, comprehensive and prospective character of these studies make them strong evidence for the safety of MMR in general (Bandolier 2002).

In response to studies of this type, which failed to substantiate the claims of anti-MMR campaigners, they retorted that 'absence of evidence is not the same as evidence of absence' (Aitken 2001b) – meaning that just because a particular study does not turn up evidence for the MMR–autism link does not prove that there is no link. (This epithet became something of a mantra.) But two things may be said in response to this. The first is that, as stated in the MCA reply to Wakefield's paper, 'it is not that there is no evidence, but that there is evidence and it does not show an association' (Arlett, Bryan 2001: 44). The second is that, if you have looked hard enough for a particular sort of evidence and have failed to find it, the sensible conclusion must be that it is not there and that it is time to think again and look elsewhere. This is how Professor Vivian Moses responded to similar demands for absolute assurances of the safety of genetically modified food products:

> Since we can judge present and future safety only on the basis of past experience, an absence of evidence of harm is precisely the only evidence we can ever expect to accumulate for the absence of harm.
>
> (Moses 2002: 2)

Alternatively, one can continue to demand that the rest of the world proves that there is no link, or one can delude oneself that the evidence really is there, if only the rest of the world could see it.

The most curious feature of the 'through a glass, darkly' paper is that it has no direct relevance to the MMR–autism link. Even if it were true that pre-licensing surveillance of MMR had been inadequate, this would not advance Dr Wakefield's claim that MMR was causing 'autistic enterocolitis' and thus contributing to an epidemic of autism. It is strange that, at a time when he was under intense pressure to substantiate this hypothesis, Dr Wakefield chose to turn aside from his own sphere of expertise (gastroenterology) to enter fields (public health and vaccination policy) in which he had no previous experience. However, a close reading of the concluding section of the paper suggests that Dr Wakefield's strategy was that, if the safety of MMR in general could be put in doubt, the credibility of any particular risk attributed to the vaccine would be raised.

Confident of finding a resonance in an increasingly risk-averse climate, Dr Wakefield invoked the 'precautionary principle' popularised by the environmentalist movement:

> Surely, when a medical intervention is intended for universal use, particularly in healthy infants, there is almost no limit to the vigilance that should be exercised.
>
> (Wakefield, Montgomery 2000: 277)

With a reference to 'healthy infants' that was guaranteed to appeal to the popular press, Dr Wakefield proposed an extreme level of caution that would deter any preventive or therapeutic intervention. In truth, there must *always* be a limit to vigilance: otherwise we allow the danger against which we are vigilant to become oppressive. Despite this, at a time when the nation was in the grip of a multiplicity of millennial anxieties, Dr Wakefield readily found the highest authority for his precautionary approach:

> As the last Minister for Health, the Hon. Frank Dobson said recently, in the context of another medical intervention, "if there is even a hypothetical risk [of harm] and a safer alternative exists, we should use it"
> (Wakefield, Montgomery 2000: 279)

As a 'precautionary measure' to prevent possible transmission of variant CJD in February 1998, Mr Dobson had insisted that albumen (derived from blood products) used as a stabiliser in some vaccines should be imported from countries not affected by BSE. If the Minister for Health himself could use a hypothetical risk to justify introducing an alternative, then so could Dr Wakefield. He argued, 'for MMR', in relation to autism and inflammatory bowel disease, 'a significant index of suspicion exists without adequate evidence of safety' (Wakefield, Montgomery 2000: 279).

Although Dr Wakefield had not clearly established either that there was 'a significant index of suspicion' about MMR or that its safety record was inadequate, his case appeared to be strengthened by coupling these two dubious propositions together. 'If the risk of chronic immune-mediated disease is increased by concurrent exposure to the component viruses of MMR, either in their natural or vaccine form' (a conditional clause that remained unvalidated), then, Dr Wakefield triumphantly concluded, by giving the vaccines separately 'we have the ability to artificially dissociate these exposures, and the possible associated risks' (Wakefield, Montgomery 2000: 279). By disparaging the safety record of MMR and inflating unsubstantiated risks, Dr Wakefield may not have advanced the MMR–autism thesis, but he had given a powerful boost to the demand for separate vaccines.

## Moving the goalposts

> If these researchers are able to prove cause and effect between immunisation and the described syndrome, they

should do so straight away. If they are unable to do so they should publicly set the matter straight lest the health of our nation's children suffers.

(Lindley, Milla 1998)

This challenge to Wakefield and his colleagues was issued by two senior gastroenterologists at Great Ormond Street Hospital for Children in immediate response to the *Lancet* paper in February 1998. Five years later Wakefield and his colleagues had still neither proven their hypothesis, nor withdrawn it.

In response to the failure of research in the two areas recommended in the *Lancet* paper – epidemiology and virology – to substantiate his hypothesis, Dr Wakefield continued to support the campaign against MMR, while redefining his case for its causative role in autism. At the outset, the concept of MMR-induced 'autistic enterocolitis' was advanced to explain a dramatic increase in the incidence of autism (the 'autism epidemic'). Before long, however, a close temporal association between MMR and the onset of behavioural regression – at first regarded as a significant indicator of causation – was relaxed and then abandoned. When epidemiological studies still failed to substantiate a link, Dr Wakefield hypothesised that MMR caused 'autistic enterocolitis' in a subset of children, rendered vulnerable by a combination of genetic and environmental factors (including food allergy, antibiotic use, ear infection, multiple concurrent vaccine exposure, a strong family history of atopic and auto-immune disease, and exposure to mercury) (Wakefield 2001b). (This list of possible cofactors in the aetiology of autism – familiar from our account of unorthodox biomedical approaches to autism – reflects Dr Wakefield's growing reliance on parent activists and anti-immunisation campaigners.)

In a response to a Danish epidemiological study (published in the *New England Journal of Medicine* in November 2002) that failed to show any link between MMR and autism, Dr Wakefield argued that this subset may be 'no more than 10 per cent of diagnoses' (Madsen et al 2002, Wakefield 2002b). In a subsequent letter to the journal, Dr Wakefield appeared to give up on epidemiology, arguing that the effect of the number and complexity of cofactors was 'to reduce statistical power to the extent that such studies fail to offer any convincing evidence either way' (Wakefield 2002b). Or as he put it in a newspaper interview in March 2003, 'retrospective studies like this are meaningless' (Phillips 2003: 43). But it was retrospective studies such as this that Wakefield specifically invited in his *Lancet* paper.

The end result of this process of shifting the goalposts is that MMR, once blamed for producing an autism epidemic, is now said to be a factor in causing autism in a number of cases too small to discern by epidemiological methods. If this is so, how can MMR have caused autism in more than 1,000 cases currently pursuing compensation under the leadership of Richard Barr (with expert medical advice from Dr Wakefield)? We know that such methods of study are capable of detecting rare adverse effects of immunisation, such as ITP at a rate of one in 32,000 vaccinations (around 20 cases a year), so detecting a subset the size of 10 per cent of all cases of autism should be fairly straightforward.

Given the failure of epidemiology to confirm his hypothesis, Dr Wakefield has counter-posed the need for clinical studies – a call loyally echoed by his anti-MMR campaign followers. But populations are made up of individuals: if an effect of MMR – a vaccine administered at a population level – cannot be discerned at a population level, then it does not exist. Furthermore, Dr Wakefield's attempts to substantiate his hypothesis at a clinical level, in collaboration with Professor O'Leary, have also failed to bear fruit.

Unfortunately, instead of accepting the failure to prove their hypothesis, and – in the interests of public health – withdrawing it, Wakefield and his supporters have doggedly and dogmatically continued to proclaim their conviction that MMR causes autism in some children, in defiance of all evidence to the contrary.

As the anti-MMR campaign found itself on the defensive, its supporters mounted increasingly personal attacks on critics of the Wakefield position. Brent Taylor and Elizabeth Miller, whose epidemiological work provided the most powerful defence of MMR, came in for particular vilification. In response to their 1999 paper, for example, Allergy-induced Autism issued a scurrilous denunciation of these authors, accusing them of 'a cynical attempt to disguise the truth' and of perpetrating 'a scandalous public dupe of BSE proportions' (AiA 1999). It demanded the resignation of 'all key members of the study group' insisting that such an 'attempt to justify health policy by using inadequate research as propaganda is reprehensible'. The criticisms of the Taylor study made by AiA were the same as those made by Dr Wakefield in a slightly more restrained letter to *The Lancet*. In his testimony to the US senate committee hearing in April 2000, Dr Wakefield claimed that the Taylor paper was the subject of a 'highly critical' debate at the Royal Statistical

Society in London, which concluded that the 'study design was wrong' (Wakefield, Montgomery 2000). In fact no such debate took place and the Royal Statistical Society came to no conclusion about the design or validity of the study. This study was described by the US Institute of Medicine's immunisation safety review as 'the most extensive epidemiological study and the strongest published evidence against the hypothesis that MMR causes ASD [austistic spectrum disorder]' (Institute of Medicine 2001: 44).

As the debate became increasingly polarised, Wakefield and his supporters resorted to impugning the motives of critics of the campaign against MMR by alleging conflicts of interest arising from their links with vaccine manufacturers. Two distinct issues thereby became confused.

First, as a result of the class action against the manufacturers of MMR, the pharmaceutical companies concerned were obliged to seek expert advice from the small pool of specialists in the relevant disciplines. These specialists received fees for their services, in the same way that expert witnesses for the plaintiffs received fees from the Legal Aid funds secured by Richard Barr and his team. Though payments should be disclosed where there is any question of a conflict of interests, the notion that the receipt of such fees implies a loss of professional discretion and integrity is both absurd and offensive. Given the low profile of pharmaceutical companies in paediatrics or autism, it is highly unlikely that any of these specialists would have become 'drug company advisors' if it were not for the activities of the anti-MMR campaign.

Second, paediatricians or immunologists who are engaged in research or clinical trials of vaccines are obliged to do this work in collaboration with pharmaceutical companies, since virtually all vaccines are manufactured by such companies. It is standard practice that researchers are excluded from investing for personal gain in companies sponsoring their research. However, although they may not gain personally, professional success is to some extent dependent upon generating research funding, so it is legitimate to declare this interest. According to Adam Finn, professor of paediatrics at the University of Bristol, such declarations should be interpreted as a qualification to give a well-informed opinion, 'as anyone unable to declare such competing interests is unlikely to have had any direct experience of using new vaccines in children' (Finn 2002: 733). However, in the rancorous climate generated by the MMR controversy, anti-MMR campaigners have presented such declarations of interest – available on easily accessible official websites – as though they were investigative journalists uncovering conspiracy and corruption. Although the implication that everybody is governed by the most venal motives is widely held in modern society, it is corrosive of any kind of civilised discourse.

Populist jibes against the drug companies are a recurrent theme among campaigners against all forms of immunisation. No doubt the pharmaceutical corporations, like all capitalist enterprises, are more concerned about their profitability than the welfare of their consumers. There are many areas in which they can be legitimately accused of profiteering, disease-mongering and sharp practice (see Moynihan et al 2002). Yet the provision of vaccines, a relatively low-volume and low-profit sector, is not one of them. Indeed it is an area characterised by low investment and declining innovation, partly as a result of the climate of risk aversion and litigiousness, particularly in the USA (Galambos 1999). In August 2003 a report by the US Institute of Medicine complained of supply problems resulting from the declining number of vaccine manufacturers and urged the government to subsidise vaccine costs (Institute of Medicine 2003). The report noted the relatively small size of the vaccine market in the USA and the fact that vaccines accounted for only 1.5% of global pharmaceutical sales. Companies complained that their return on investment was small and there was little incentive towards research and development. In a contribution to a conference on vaccination in the USA in October 2003, Richard Gallagher, editor of *The Scientist*, noted that 'vaccinations are unattractive targets for industry, under-appreciated from the public health perspective, under-funded by basic research organisations, and treated with suspicion by the public' (Gallagher 2003). He commented on the 'malign influence' of three groups – anti-vaccination lobbyists (whose 'ignorant' websites included contributions from 'health nuts, conspiracy theorists and misguided physicians'), journalists (who wrote 'badly-researched and poorly-argued scare stories') and lawyers. At the same conference, vaccine specialist Neil Halsey noted that class action lawsuits led to large damage awards and complained that the courts provided a forum for 'junk science' in the guise of expert testimony (*The Daily News*, 27 October 2003).

# 9

# MISSING LINKS

It is my impression that the trend in autism incidence is
wholly consistent with a causal relationship with the MMR
vaccine at the population level.
(Testimony of Dr Andrew Wakefield before
the Government Reform Committee, US House
of Representatives, 25 April 2001;
Wakefield 2001b: 10)

There are four links in the proposed chain of causality connecting
MMR to autism:

1. MMR immunisation leads to chronic measles infection (and
   immune dysfunction).
2. 'Autistic Enterocolitis'/'New-Variant Inflammatory Bowel
   Disease' results from measles infection.
3. 'Leaky Bowel' (resulting from 'Autistic Enterocolitis'/'New-
   Variant Inflammatory Bowel Disease') allows toxic opioid
   peptides to enter the bloodstream.
4. 'Opioid excess' causes 'regressive' or 'atypical' autism.

Let us look at each of these links in turn.

## Does MMR cause measles?

The first requirement of the MMR–autism hypothesis is that MMR
immunisation results in chronic measles infection in some children.
Those who believe that it does, often also express concern that of the
combination of immunisations against three distinct diseases in the
MMR vaccination results in a damaging overload or suppression of
the infantile immune system.

The MMR vaccine contains an 'attenuated' strain of the measles virus. This means that it has been specially developed to diminish its capacity to cause disease, while conserving its capacity to provoke an antibody reaction that will protect against further exposure to the wild measles virus. The MMR–autism hypothesis suggests that the attenuated strain of measles in MMR in some way produces a chronic measles infection, which may affect the gastrointestinal tract or the central nervous system (or both). The three viruses in MMR are all RNA viruses, which are much smaller and less stable than DNA viruses, such as those causing herpes or chickenpox. As anybody who has suffered from recurrent cold sores or shingles can testify, these viruses can persist in a latent form in the human body for life. By contrast, RNA viruses need to replicate to survive and nobody has yet identified any site at which either the wild or vaccine strains of these viruses can persist for more than a few weeks. (The persistence of the measles virus in cases of the rare condition SSPE [see below] is the only known, and still unexplained, exception.)

It is well recognised that MMR may produce minor adverse reactions: malaise, fever, rash and, occasionally, fever fits (febrile convulsions) and parotid swelling (like mumps). Although diarrhoea and vomiting have been recorded as 'undesirable effects' noted in the six weeks following MMR, they have not been identified as a persistent feature. More rarely, MMR can cause joint pains and swellings and a blood disorder associated with a rash (idiopathic thrombocytopenic purpura; ITP), which usually resolves spontaneously. Like any immunisation, MMR can very rarely provoke an acute allergic (anaphylactic) reaction: in the USA since 1990, some 70 million measles vaccinations have resulted in 11 cases of anaphylaxis (none fatal). But none of these reactions suggests an ongoing measles infection.

There has been much controversy over whether measles immunisation (either separately, or in the forms of MR and MMR) can cause encephalitis – an inflammation of the brain that occurs in measles itself at a rate of around one in 1,000 cases. A number of studies have investigated this possibility (Bedford, Elliman 2001). The biggest population studied was the 7 million British children who received the MR immunisation in 1994. Of the 11 cases of encephalitis attributed to MR, a definite diagnosis was made in six. Ten made a complete recovery and one child was left with residual paralysis, but, as there was no change in his measles antibody level, it was considered unlikely that the vaccination caused this condition.

There is thus considerable doubt whether measles vaccination ever causes encephalitis; if it does, it does so at a rate of less than one in a million doses (at least one thousand times less than measles itself).

Subacute sclerosing pan-encephalitis (SSPE) is a rare but devastating complication that occurs at a rate of around one in 100,000 cases of measles. A progressive and invariably fatal neurodegenerative disorder, it begins several years after infection, although the pathology of the condition is not fully understood. The incidence of SSPE has been dramatically reduced by measles and MMR immunisation and it has now virtually disappeared in developed countries. Neither measles nor MMR immunisations have ever been shown to cause SSPE; one case occurred following the MR campaign in Britain, but investigation confirmed that it was caused by wild measles virus rather than by the vaccine.

If MMR causes inflammatory bowel disease or autism, it would appear to do so without producing any intermediate manifestations of measles infection, either in the bowel or the brain. But what about the effects of MMR on the immune system?

The suggestion that giving three vaccines simultaneously is too much for the infantile immune system was investigated by the US vaccine specialist Paul Offit and colleagues (Offit et al 2002). The researchers point out that, although we give infants more vaccines today than in the past, the higher quality of the vaccines means that the number of antigens they receive has declined. For example, the old smallpox vaccine, which was used until smallpox was eradicated in the 1970s, contained 200 proteins. Now the 11 vaccines routinely administered in the USA contain fewer than 130 proteins (and more than half of these are in the chickenpox vaccine that has yet to be introduced in Britain). They also calculate that the infant immune system has the theoretical capacity to respond to 'about 10,000 vaccines at any one time'. Put another way, they reckon that, if all 11 vaccines were given at the same time, 'then about 0.1% of the immune system would be "used up"' (Offit et al 2002: 126). They insist that 'young infants have an enormous capacity to respond to multiple vaccines, as well as to the many other challenges present in the environment'.

In Britain, a team led by Dr Elizabeth Miller at the Public Health Laboratory Service (and including Royal Free community paediatrician Brent Taylor) found another method of assessing the impact of MMR on the immune system (Miller et al 2003). They hypothesised that 'if MMR vaccine does induce clinically significant immunosuppression, susceptibility to infection should be increased in the post-vaccination period'. They tested this hypothesis using cases of invasive bacterial infection and pneumonia in children between 12 and 23 months admitted to hospital over a four-year period in selected districts in the Thames region. They found that there was no increased risk of hospitalisation with such infections within three months of vaccination; indeed, there was a slight protective effect. They concluded that their results provided 'no support for the concept of "immunological overload" induced by multiple antigen vaccinations, nor calls for single antigen vaccines' (Miller et al 2003: 222).

Dr Offit has also challenged the notion that measles immunisation is more likely to provoke an auto-immune response than natural measles infection (Offit 2000). He points out that during natural measles infection the virus reproduces rapidly causing disease and provoking an immune response. By contrast, the attenuated strain in the vaccine reproduces sluggishly, does not cause disease and provokes a much lower immune response. Because the immune response is much greater after natural infection, this should also produce a greater auto-immune response:

> If this were the case, then autoimmunity should occur *more* frequently after natural infection than after vaccination. Or, said another way, if measles virus caused autism, measles vaccination would *lower*, not raise, the incidence of autism.
>
> (Offit 2000: 2, emphasis in original)

### 'New variant' inflammatory bowel disease?

The next link in the chain is the new diagnostic entity identified in the February 1998 *Lancet* paper: 'autistic enterocolitis', later dubbed by Dr Wakefield 'new variant' inflammatory bowel disease (Wakefield et al 2000). The characteristic features of this condition were said to be the presence of enlarged patches of lymphatic tissue, particularly around the lower end of the small intestine ('ileal lymphoid-nodular hyperplasia'; ILNH) and inflammation of the lining (mucosa) of both the small and large bowel (enterocolitis).

There are a number of areas of controversy surrounding this condition, the existence of which is still not generally accepted either among gastroenterologists or among autism specialists. The first arises from Dr Wakefield's earlier work on the relationship between measles and inflammatory bowel disease (IBD). The second concerns the question of whether the findings suggestive of inflammation reported in the *Lancet* paper are specific to children with developmental disorder, as Dr Wakefield's team maintains. (A third, the question of whether measles virus – wild or vaccine strain – has been identified in specimens from the guts of autistic children, was considered in Chapter 8).

In 1993 Dr Wakefield first claimed to have detected evidence of persistent measles infection in patients with Crohn's disease (Wakefield et al 1993). Further researches (including some by other members of the Royal Free group) using more sensitive techniques have failed to confirm the measles–IBD link (Afzal, 1998a, 1998b, Chadwick et al, 1998). The American Academy of Pediatrics review commented that 'variations in methodology could explain some of the discrepancies in reported results from the different laboratories studying intestinal biopsy specimens' (Halsey 2001: 24). This review also observed that 'false positive results in highly capable laboratories have led to incorrect conclusions about infectious agents causing many chronic diseases, including multiple sclerosis and schizophrenia' (Halsey 2001: 24). Measles, in particular, has been implicated in Paget's disease of the bone, diabetes and systemic lupus erythematosus, as well as multiple sclerosis and Crohn's disease.

In 1998 the World Health Organization reviewed the biological, microbiological and epidemiological evidence and concluded that it did not support a link between measles virus infection or vaccine and IBD (Metcalf 1998, WHO 1998). It is curious that, at around the time that further researches were failing to confirm a link between measles virus and IBD, Dr Wakefield appears to have developed the MMR–autism hypothesis, which assumes the existence of this link.

What about the appearance of gut inflammation in autistic children that seemed to have so impressed the Royal Free team? There was considerable dispute over the significance of the colonoscopy findings reported in Wakefield's *Lancet* paper. Two gastroenterologists from Great Ormond Street Hospital for Children in London insisted, on the basis of 329 consecutive colonoscopies, that 'chronic non-specific colitis, as described by Wakefield, is a common form of non-infective colonic inflammation in the age group studied' (Lindley, Milla 1998: 907). They further noted that 85 per cent of these children had minor immuno-deficiencies, but none had a neuropsychiatric disorder. Earlier research suggested that lymphoid nodular hyperplasia (LNH) (for Wakefield the key feature of 'autistic enterocolitis') was a common and benign condition that disappeared spontaneously, with no long-term consequences. Indeed, critics cited an earlier paper by Professor John Walker-Smith, a co-author of the *Lancet* paper, which described LNH as benign 'due to the frequency of its demonstration in asymptomatic children' (although Walker-Smith has disputed this interpretation of his work).

In subsequent papers Dr Wakefield and his team attempted to clarify the distinctive pathological features of autistic enterocolitis. In their study of 60 children (including the *Lancet* 12), they found LNH in the ileum in 93 per cent of children with developmental disorder, and signs of chronic colitis in 88 per cent (Wakefield et al 2000). The authors described the mucosal inflammation as 'mild to moderate' in character, characterising it as 'a subtle new variant of IBD that lacks the specific diagnostic features of either Crohn's disease . . . or ulcerative colitis' (Wakefield et al 2000: 2293). A further paper provided more detailed analysis of 21 cases of 'autistic enterocolitis', confirming that it was 'endoscopically and histologically subtle' (Furlano et al 2001). However, as with the 1998 *Lancet* report, problems of selection bias and inadequate controls made it difficult to draw conclusions from these studies. The 2001 Medical Research Council review advised that 'caution must be exercised in extrapolating from results seen in children referred to a paediatric gastroenterology unit' (MRC 2001: 34). It also suggested that 'the most informative control groups, children matched for abnormal eating behaviour and/or degree of constipation, should have been investigated' (MRC 2001: 34).

Dr Wakefield and his supporters have cited a number of studies to substantiate their 'autistic enterocolitis' thesis. A group of researchers in Washington DC wrote to *The Lancet* in response to the February 1998 paper indicating their enthusiasm for the concept of ILNH, which they had noted in children with food allergies (and other manifestations of atopy) (Sabra et al 1998). In particular they had found ILNH in two children with food allergies and attention deficit hyperactivity disorder (ADHD), and they believed that this mediated between the digestive and behavioural problems. Although this research has been widely quoted by Dr Wakefield and his supporters, it is worth noting that it has not been published in any fuller form than this short letter, that it is based on two cases, and that it links food allergy and ADHD (rather than MMR and autism). Although it does confirm that another group of researchers have also seen ILNH, Professor Walker-Smith may have been overstating the significance of this study when he claimed that this letter is a 'great public vindication' of the Royal Free team and 'our whole concept of ILNH' (Walker-Smith 2003: 244).

Another frequently cited study is that by Karoly Horvath and his team at the University of Maryland. Dr Horvath – known for his earlier endorsement of secretin (see Chapter 6) – conducted endoscopic examinations of the upper gastro-intestinal tracts of 36 children with autism (Horvath et al 1999). He found that 70 per cent had signs of inflammation of the gullet resulting from stomach acid ('reflux oesophagitis'), while a smaller proportion also had inflammation of the stomach and first part of the small intestine ('gastritis and duodenitis'). Apart from suggesting that a number of autistic children may have problems in the upper as well as the lower digestive tract, these findings add nothing to the controversy about autistic enterocolitis.

The findings of two groups of researchers sympathetic to the Wakefield campaign have been disclosed to the public and widely circulated on the Internet. In endoscopies carried out on more than 100 children with autism, Dr Tim Buie, a paediatric gastroenterologist in Boston, has identified LNH in 16 per cent and colitis (not Crohn's disease or ulcerative colitis) in 12 per cent (Buie et al 2002). He has claimed that 'more than 50 per cent of autistic children appear to have gastrointestinal symptoms, food allergies, and maldigestion or malabsorption issues' (Buie et al 2002: 1). Though Dr Buie has presented these findings at conferences attended by parents of autistic children in Portland in November 2001, in San Diego in October 2002 and in Chicago in May 2003, by the end of 2003 they had still not been published in a form in which they can be properly evaluated. In a similar way, Dr Arthur Krigsman of New York presented 'preliminary data' at a congressional hearing in June 2002 (Krigsman 2002). He found enterocolitis in 65 per cent of 43 patients with autism and LNH in 90 per cent. The fact that, nearly two years later, this study remains unpublished means that it is impossible to draw any definite conclusions. The premature disclosure of unvalidated scientific researches to the public, also noted in Chapter 8, has become a consistent feature of the anti-MMR campaign.

## Leaky bowel?

The third link in the causal chain purported between MMR and autism is the notion of a 'leaky bowel'. The Wakefield hypothesis suggests that inflammation, secondary to chronic measles infection, renders the bowel lining (mucosa) more permeable to opioid peptides, which enter the circulation in excessive quantities. It is generally recognised that there has been very little research in this area, and the available evidence is largely indirect. One frequently quoted study found increased gut permeability to sugars in nine out of 21 patients with autism (D'Eufemia 1996). But, even allowing for the small size of this sample and the unconfirmed nature of the results, the fact that sugars are much smaller molecules than proteins or peptides means that it is of doubtful significance in relation to the passage of opioid peptides – a point acknowledged by Dr Wakefield in 2002 (Wakefield 2002) (although not in the reference to this work in his 1998 *Lancet* paper).

In the absence of evidence on the specific question of the effect on gut permeability to peptides of autistic enterocolitis, Dr Wakefield fell back on a range of other 'by no means mutually exclusive hypotheses for the *liaison dangereuse* between gut and brain' (Wakefield 2002). One such hypothesis is that autism results from 'gut flora dysbiosis', from excessive growths of various bacteria, yeasts and other organisms, from which toxins pass through the bowel lining and enter the bloodstream. There have been claims of therapeutic benefit from the treatment of *Clostridium tetani* with vancomycin (an antibiotic which is not absorbed from the gut) and from measures to eradicate candida (thrush). According to the Medical Research Council's 2001 review of autism research, this is 'an area where speculation currently outweighs published literature' (MRC 2001: 36).

Another hypothesis that has also been invoked by Dr Wakefield and his supporters is the 'impaired sulphation' theory advanced by the biochemist Dr Rosemary Waring and her colleagues in Birmingham, England. According to this theory, children with autism have an impairment of the mechanism for sulphate metabolism, which could result in increased intestinal permeability. The MRC review considered that this theory was 'potentially biologically plausible but remains unproven'. It was concerned that published data came only from Waring's group, using indirect assay methods and indicated the need for 'independent replication of these findings', preferably using more direct methods (MRC 2001: 37). But, even if these hypotheses, and others, are not incompatible with the MMR–autism hypothesis, it does not mean that they support it.

The most comprehensive critique of the 'leaky bowel' thesis comes from New York neurobiologist Michael Gershon (Gershon 2001). Professor Gershon concedes that it is plausible that inflammation could result in increased permeability of the lining of the bowel. However, peptides are too large to cross cell membranes and must go through the 'paracellular' pathway in between cells. But, if this pathway is open to molecules passing from the cavity of the intestine into the tissue of the body, then it must also allow the passage of molecules from the body into the bowel. As Gershon puts it, 'if the presumed "leak" were large enough to permit peptides to enter the body in significant amounts, then body proteins would be expected to move simultaneously in the opposite direction into the lumen of the bowel' (Gershon 2001: 3). However, the phenomenon of 'protein-losing enteropathy', although recognised in other conditions, has never been reported in association with autism or with MMR.

Gershon acknowledges the possibility that a putative measles infection produces a selective leak, which might allow opioid peptides to enter, but not allow the larger-body protein molecules to exit. However, any such mechanism would disrupt other molecular transport mechanisms and cause malnutrition, again, not a recognised feature of autism. Another question also arises: why do children who suffer from inflammatory bowel disease or immune deficiency states, whose guts are known to be 'leaky', not develop autism or other neuropsychiatric syndromes?

Gershon also points out that the notion of a 'leaky bowel' allowing toxic peptides to enter the bloodstream and to damage the brain neglects two other important defence mechanisms: the liver and the 'blood–brain barrier'. Blood from the gut passes directly to the liver, which plays the role of a filter: 'opiates, in particular, are detoxified in the liver'. There has been no suggestion that liver function is abnormal in children with autism, or indeed, following MMR. The blood–brain barrier evolved to protect the brain from potential toxins circulating in the bloodstream and relatively large molecules such as peptides are unable to cross (unless they have some specialised transport mechanism). For a gut-derived peptide to cause autism, says Gershon, it requires 'that a miracle occurs to cause the blood–brain barrier to open, like the Red Sea did for Moses and the Israelites during their exodus from Egypt' (Gershon 2001: 5).

Furthermore, Gershon argues that there is no reason to invoke such an implausible biological pathway to explain the association of bowel disturbance with autism. The nervous system of the gut (Gershon's specialist interest) resembles the brain in its structure and in the role of hormones and neurotransmitters: 'The brain can thus disturb the gut and the gut can disturb the brain; both might equally be abnormal for whatever the genetic reason for autism turns out to be' (Gershon 2001: 6).

## Opioid excess?

The final link in the MMR–autism chain of causality is the opioid excess theory, which was discussed in Chapter 6. If proponents of this theory are asked how they think opioid peptides produce autistic behaviour, they tend to resort to a combination of argument by analogy and speculation (this is, of course, how the opioid excess theory arose in the first place).

Because of their conviction that some children are born autistic (as a result of some combination of genes and intrauterine or peri-natal pathology) and that others undergo autistic regression (as a result of exposure to MMR and/or other presumed toxins), advo-cates of the opioid excess theory have attempted to use this frame-work to explain both processes. They argue that opioids are teratogenic in the developing fetus and encephalopathic in the infant. The teratogenic theory is that during pregnancy, opioid pep-tides pass from the mother's gut into her bloodstream and thence via the placenta into the fetus, where, at a particular stage of develop-ment, they cause the neurological damage that results in autism. The encephalopathic theory is that during infancy immunisation with MMR causes autistic enterocolitis, which allows opioid peptides to pass into the child's circulation and thence through the blood–brain barrier to cause brain damage resulting in the characteristic features of regressive autism, now redefined as a 'subacute encephalopathy' (Wakefield 2002).

The main argument for both mechanisms is an analogy. The effect of opioid peptides on the developing fetus is said to be analogous to that of drugs such as thalidomide or sodium valproate, both of which have been shown to cause fetal brain damage resulting in autism. The effect of opioid peptides on the infant brain is said to be analogous to the encephalopathy that results from liver failure. First suggested by Dr Wakefield in a paper in 2000, the hepatic encephalopathy model was further developed in a 2002 review article (Wakefield 2000, 2002). However, an analogy suggests superficial similarities: closer analysis may reveal that the differences are more significant. Drugs may be toxic to the developing fetus, but there is no evidence that maternal diet contributes to the development of autism. Nor is there any evidence that mothers with inflammatory bowel disease, who might be expected by Dr Wakefield to have increased gut permeability to opioid peptides, have an increased risk of bearing babies with autism. The encephalopathy associated with advanced liver disease causes confusion and impaired consciousness, it is progressive if not treated, and reversible if treated: none of these features in typical autism.

As a result of his reliance on analogy, Dr Wakefield's MMR–autism hypothesis has become increasingly diffuse and the causal links increasingly tenuous. To a critical eye it appears that, in the hope of finding any shred of support for his theory, he has primed a computer search engine with the combination of the categories 'any gut abnormality' and 'any psychiatric disorder'. For example, in the most recent and most comprehensive account of his hypothesis, he asserts that 'constipation alone may precipitate acute confusional states in the elderly', as though this statement in some way supports his MMR–autism thesis (Wakefield et al 2002: 664). We have seen above how Dr Wakefield welcomed the support of Sabra et al, who linked food allergy to ADHD. He also points to a link between undiagnosed coeliac disease (gluten enteropathy) and 'behavioural disturbances, with a tendency to depression, irritability and impaired school performance' (Wakefield et al 2002: 664)[1]. But coeliac disease is not IBD, and a bad day at school is not autism. Furthermore people with coeliac disease are not more likely to be autistic and people who are autistic are not more likely to have coeliac disease.

As Dr Wakefield spreads his net wider and wider to incorporate alternative theories of autism, his own becomes increasingly attenuated. Thus, when he brings in theories of gut dysbiosis, impaired sulphation or heavy metal toxicity, MMR recedes into the background. At the other end of the chain, autism has to take its place alongside ADHD, depression, hepatic encephalopathy and schizophrenia. There is a serious danger that, if the histology of autistic entero-

---

1   In his *Lancet* paper, Dr Wakefield claims that 'Asperger first recorded the link between coeliac disease and behavioural psychoses' (Wakefield et al 1998: 639). He provides a reference (misspelled, with incorrect page numbers) to a paper published in German in 1961 (Asperger 1961). Dr Wakefield here echoes Mary Coleman's comment that 'Coeliac disease was first reported by Asperger in 1961 in patients with his syndrome' (Coleman 1997: 219) (she provides the same incorrect reference). In fact, Asperger's paper, which reports a follow-up study carried out on 12 children with coeliac disease, makes no mention of 'behavioural psychoses', or autism or Asperger's syndrome. It simply discusses a range of psychological problems observed in children with coeliac disease.

colitis becomes any more subtle, the whole chain of causality will simply disintegrate.

While evidence for the MMR–autism hypothesis has proved elusive, Dr Wakefield's speculations have become increasingly imaginative. In his 2002 review he cited a European patent application that claims to have identified more neuropeptides in the urine of autistic children. These include dermophine, described as a 'potent hallucinogen':

> In nature, it is found in the skin of non-captive South American poison dart frogs, where it may be a microbial product, providing possible clues to its origin in the urine of autistic children.
>
> (Wakefield et al 2002: 668)

If you think that the behaviour of autistic children is 'a bit like' that of wild rainforest frogs on acid, then you might think that this is a thesis worth exploring.

## Epidemiology

Further epidemiological studies have attempted to test the shifting terms of Dr Wakefield's MMR–autism hypothesis. As reported in Chapter 8, one of Dr Wakefield's objections to Brent Taylor's 1999 study was that it had not considered children who had received MMR at any age, and developed autism at any time after immunisation (although Wakefield's *Lancet* paper had emphasised a close temporal association, on average, less than one week). Professor Taylor and his colleagues conducted a further study to answer this question. Their results showed no increased risk of autism after MMR immunisation, whether given as primary immunisation, as a booster dose or as part of a catch-up exercise shortly after MMR immunisation was introduced in 1988 (Farrington et al 2001).

When Dr Wakefield suggested that a failure to take account of a range of co-factors explained the failure of epidemiological studies to confirm the emergence of a 'new variant' form of autism, Professor Taylor and colleagues isolated two requirements of the new hypothesis:

- The proportion of autistic children with regression and bowel symptoms should be higher in those children who were given

MMR before parents became concerned about their development.
• The pattern of bowel problems and regression in autism should have changed after MMR was introduced.

They returned to their study population to examine these questions, and found that:

• The proportion of children with autism who had developmental regression or bowel problems had not changed over two decades since 1979.
• Neither developmental regression nor bowel problems in children with autism were associated with MMR vaccination.
• There was no evidence for a 'new variant' form of autism. (Taylor et al 2002)

This study made another significant finding: a review of records showed that in the cases of 13 children the history given by the parents had changed after the extensive publicity about the link between MMR and autism. Whereas parents had previously reported concerns before their child's first birthday, they now recorded symptoms as developing only after MMR vaccination, in some cases shortly after.

A number of other epidemiological studies have also failed to confirm an association between MMR and autism.

James Kaye and colleagues studied the cases of 305 children diagnosed with autism between 1988 and 1999, and who were included in the UK general practice research database (Kaye et al 2001). They found a sevenfold increase in the incidence of autism over this period, during which the uptake of MMR was virtually constant at 95 per cent. There was no time correlation between the prevalence of MMR vaccination and the incidence of autism, strong evidence against a causal association.

Another study in general practice in Britain inquired whether children who went on to be diagnosed as autistic consulted their GPs more often than other children in the six months following MMR (DeWilde et al 2001). They found that there was no difference in consulting behaviour in autistic children compared with controls.

Loring Dales and colleagues identified autistic children born between 1980 and 1994 from the California Department of Development Services and collected data on MMR immunisation from the California Department of Health Services (Dales et al

2001). They found a 373 per cent increase in the incidence of autism over this period, but only a 14 per cent increase in uptake of MMR. They concluded that MMR could not explain the increasing incidence of autism.

Eric Fombonne, an autism specialist and epidemiologist formerly at the Maudsley Hospital in London and now in Montreal, and Suniti Chakrabarti, community paediatrician in Stafford, England, tested Wakefield's MMR–autism hypothesis using 'the Stafford sample' – children with a diagnosis of autism born between 1992 and 1995 (Fombonne, Chakrabarti 2001). These children were compared with the Maudsley Hospital Clinical sample – children with autism born since 1987, who had received MMR – and with the Maudsley Family Study sample – children with autism born before 1979, who had not had MMR. This approach overcomes the problems of selection bias in the Royal Free studies. These researchers looked at the age at which parents became concerned about their child's behaviour and found that, on average, this was at around 19 months, whether or not the child had received MMR. Furthermore, there was no difference in the proportion of children who experienced developmental regression in the groups that had received MMR and those that had not. Of the 96 children in the Stafford sample, none was found to have an inflammatory bowel disorder. No association was found between developmental regression and gastro-intestinal symptoms. The authors concluded that 'no evidence was found to support a distinct syndrome of MMR-induced autism or of "autistic enterocolitis"' (Fombonne, Chakrabarti 2001: 1). They indicated that two important messages emerged from their study. The first was that there was no evidence to justify any change in immunisation policy. The second was that:

> It should no longer be acceptable that investigators who still argue for a MMR–autism link fail to provide precise and replicable clinical and developmental data on their autism samples, thereby maintaining a degree of ambiguity and confusion that is damaging to both the public health and the science.
>
> (Fombonne and Chakrabarti 2001: 7)

In addition to the Finnish studies noted in Chapter 8, studies from other Scandinavian countries added to the weight of epidemiological evidence against the Wakefield hypothesis. These studies are particularly reliable because these countries have long-established immunisation programmes, relatively stable populations, and high quality health and public records. In Sweden, Professor Christopher Gillberg and Dr Harald Heijbel re-analysed the data from a population study of autism performed in the late 1980s (Gillberg, Heijbel 1998). They divided cases of autism into those who were born before the introduction of MMR and those born later who had received MMR, but they found that there was no increased risk of developing autism in the latter group. They concluded that this study did not support the hypothesis of an association between MMR and autistic disorder. They also looked at cases of 'atypical autism' and found that these also showed no association with MMR.

In Denmark, Madsen and colleagues undertook a retrospective cohort study of all children born in Denmark from 1991 to 1998, a total of 537,303, of whom 82 per cent had received MMR (Madsen et al 2002). They identified 316 children with autism and another 422 with an autistic spectrum disorder. The relative risk of autism in the vaccinated children, compared with the unvaccinated group, was 0.92; the relative risk of another autistic spectrum disorder was 0.83. In other words, the risk of autism was similar in children who had received MMR and those who had not. They found that there was no association between age at the time of vaccination, the time since vaccination or the date of vaccination, and the development of autistic disorder. They concluded that this provided strong evidence against the MMR–autism hypothesis.

## Expert reviews

Given the potential importance of Dr Wakefield's claims and the consequences for immunisation policy if they were valid, a number of agencies convened expert inquiries to examine his work. These included the Medical Research Council (MRC) in Britain, the American Academy of Pediatrics and the US Institute of Medicine Committee on Immunisation Safety. Supporters of the anti-MMR campaign often give the impression that the Wakefield case has been suppressed, not given a fair hearing, or that it has been summarily dismissed by politicians or bureaucrats. A brief survey shows that Dr Wakefield's work has been subjected to serious scrutiny by some of the leading experts in the relevant academic and clinical disciplines, not only in Britain but in the USA (and in other countries). If there has been any resistance to a full discussion it has come from Dr Wakefield and his supporters.

## The Medical Research Council

Following its one-day *ad hoc* review of Dr Wakefield's case in March 1998 and the March 2000 report of its expert subgroup, in March 2001 the MRC was commissioned by the Department of Health to review the current state of research on the epidemiology and causes of autism. The review was chaired by the Edinburgh psychiatrist Professor Eve Johnstone, who coordinated four subgroups. Three groups were of scientists and the fourth was a lay group, which included parent activists, such as Rosemary Kessick of Allergy-induced Autism and Jonathan Tommey of *The Autism File*, as well as prominent figures from the National Autistic Society. Although Dr Wakefield was invited to attend the review or to make a submission to it, he declined on the grounds that several of its members had been retained by the defendants (vaccine manufacturers) in the impending MMR litigation and hence had a conflict of interest. Professor O'Leary is recorded as having made no response to an invitation from the inquiry. A 91-page report was published in December 2001 (MRC 2001).

From the outset the MRC review was concerned that public debate about autism had focused almost exclusively on the suggested link with MMR. Considering there was little more to add to the earlier MRC reports on this subject, this review sought to investigate broader questions about the causes of autistic spectrum disorders and the controversy surrounding the apparent increase in the incidence of these conditions. However, the lay group posed this question:

> Does further evidence published since the last MRC review and specifically examining possible associations between MMR and autistic spectrum disorders (ASDs) alter the conclusions of that review?
>
> (MRC 2001: 28)

In response, the experts concluded that 'the current epidemiological evidence does not support the proposed link of MMR to ASDs' (MRC 2001: 31). Under considerable pressure from lay group members strongly committed to the MMR link, the review conceded that there remained a 'theoretical possibility' that MMR could contribute to autism in a small number of children. The report emphasised that 'more extensive research would be necessary to provide evidence for the biological plausibility of a suggested causal link between viral infections and ASDs (as this is currently not robust), as it would be for other proposed causal factors' (MRC 2001: 28).

The review considered a range of factors that have been implicated as causes of autism (and as pointers towards interventions), particularly by proponents of unorthodox biomedical theories. These include mercury, lead, dietary factors (casein, gluten, etc), gut flora dysbiosis, disordered sulphur metabolism and immune dysfunction, neurotransmitter theories. The common theme was a plethora of claims either not substantiated or contradicted by other researchers, often published in the 'grey literature' without adequate peer review or quality control. The report proposed further research in all these areas, emphasising that 'greater methodological rigour and independent replication are crucial' (MRC 2001:52).

### The American Academy of Pediatrics

The American Academy of Pediatrics (AAP) convened a two-day conference in June 2000 in Oak Brook, Illinois, at which 'parents, practitioners and scientists presented information and research on MMR vaccine and ASD'. An expert panel reviewed videotaped testimony by Dr Wakefield and Professor O'Leary from the congressional committee hearings in April 2000, and a further written submission from Dr Wakefield. (Dr Wakefield complained that 'the original meeting was rescheduled for a date that made it impossible for Professor O'Leary and I to attend' [Wakefield 2001a].)

The panel responded to the question 'Does the available evidence support a causal relationship between MMR vaccine and the pathogenesis of autistic spectrum disorders (ASD)?' by applying formal causality criteria: strength of association, consistency, specificity, temporality, biological gradient, plausibility, coherence, experimental evidence, and analogy ('the weakest form of evidence for a causal argument'). The conclusion of the panel's 42-page report was unequivocal: 'the available evidence does not support the hypothesis that MMR vaccine causes autism or associated disorders or IBD' (Halsey 2001: 29). The AAP rejected the call for separate vaccines and urged paediatricians to continue to promote the childhood immunisation programme and further research into the causes of ASDs.

## *Institute of Medicine, Committee on Immunisation Safety*

In response to continuing publicity in the USA about the MMR–autism link, the Center for Disease Control and the National Institute of Health asked the Institute of Medicine to set up a independent committee on immunisation to review this matter (McCormick 2001). In January 2001 it convened a 15-strong committee including experts in the relevant fields, which reviewed the literature and held an open meeting attended by academic researchers, government scientists, federal officials and representatives of vaccine safety advocacy groups. It sought presentations of both published and unpublished work from those actively engaged in research in this area. Dr Wakefield did not attend, complaining that 'unfortunately due to the presence of the press, virological data undergoing peer review, could not be presented, which largely defeated the purpose of the meeting' (Wakefield 2001a). A working group of the committee conferred with parents of autistic children as well as with vaccine safety advocates. The committee's 69-page report was published in April 2001 (Institute of Medicine 2001).

The committee's conclusion was that 'the evidence favours rejection of a causal relationship at the population level between MMR vaccine and ASD'. It cited the following evidence:

A consistent body of epidemiological evidence shows no association at a population level between MMR vaccine and ASD;

The original case series of children with ASD and bowel symptoms and other available case reports are uninformative with respect to causality;

Biological models linking MMR vaccine and ASD are fragmentary;

There is no relevant animal model linking MMR vaccine and ASD.

(Institute of Medicine 2001: 46)

The committee added a significant caveat. It indicated that its conclusion did 'not exclude the possibility that MMR vaccine could contribute to ASD in a small number of children', because the epidemiological evidence lacked the precision to assess such rare occurrences. Furthermore, 'the proposed biological models linking MMR vaccine to ASD, although far from established, are nevertheless not disproved' (Institute of Medicine 2001: 46).

The anti-MMR campaign leapt on these sentences – which have been repeated in various forms in subsequent inquiries – insisting that 'the jury is still out'; epidemiology is a 'blunt tool'; 'more research needs to be done'. Yet this statement does no more than state a truism: it is impossible to prove a negative. However, the pursuit of an increasingly small effect, in the face of mounting evidence that it does not exist, cannot be regarded as a rational deployment of scarce research funds.

# 10

# THE METAMORPHOSIS OF ANDREW WAKEFIELD

He is tall, handsome, fluent, charismatic and above all a man of conviction. He is a man of utter sincerity and honesty. In reality the out-of-fashion term 'crusader after truth' would best describe him.

> (Dr Wakefield as described by Professor John Walker-Smith; Walker-Smith 2003: 242)

He's got a good sense of humour, cultured British accent, good looks and the body of a rugby player.

> (Spectrum Interview 2000)

We are in the midst of an international epidemic. Those responsible for investigating and dealing with this epidemic have failed. Among the reasons for this failure is the fact that they are faced with the prospect that they themselves may be responsible for the epidemic. Therefore, in their attempts to exonerate themselves they are an impediment to progress. I believe that public health officials know that there is a problem; they are, however, willing to deny the problem and accept the loss of an unknown number of children on the basis that the success of public health policy – mandatory vaccination – by necessity involves sacrifice.

> (Dr Wakefield's address to 'Power of One Idea' rally, Washington DC, 22 April 2002 (at www.whale.to/vaccines/wakefield.htm).

Dr Wakefield has become a pivotal figure for many in the parents' campaign; a handsome, glossy-haired charismatic hero to families of autistic children in this country and America . . . It's not hard to imagine Russell Crowe playing

Dr Wakefield opposite Julia Roberts as a feisty single mother fighting for justice for her child.
(Justine Picardie, *The Telegraph Magazine*, 8 June 2002)

'Hello, I'm Andy'. Dr Wakefield (Hugh Bonneville) introduces himself as the caring, listening doctor to Nicky (Jamie Martin) – a little boy with autism – and his mother Christine (Juliet Stevenson), in *Hear the Silence*, Channel Five's dramatisation of the MMR–autism story, screened 15 December 2003.

Dr Wakefield, the central personality in the MMR story, emerges as a tragic figure. At the outset, he appeared as a serious scientific researcher. Following the publication of the *Lancet* paper, he rapidly acquired the reputation of maverick defying the medical, and political, establishment. Although he was feted as a hero by some parents of autistic children and anti-immunisation activists, he became increasingly alienated from the world of medical science.

When, in December 2001 Dr Wakefield resigned from the Royal Free, to a substantial section of public opinion the crusader appeared as a martyr to medical orthodoxy. When he announced his acceptance of a post at a privately-funded research centre in Florida, to many in the medical world it seemed that a promising career had reached a premature end.

## The listening doctor

Although Dr Wakefield has become widely known for his MMR–autism hypothesis he has no background in immunisation or child psychiatry, indeed, he is not a paediatrician. After postgraduate training in surgery, he carried out research in small bowel transplantation in Canada in the mid-1980s. He subsequently switched from surgery to medical gastroenterology, and returned to Britain to pursue research in inflammatory bowel diseases (such as Crohn's disease and ulcerative colitis) at the Royal Free. In 1989 he published a well-received paper on 'the pathogenesis of Crohn's disease', proposing that the characteristic features of this condition arose from areas of tissue damage caused by loss of blood supply resulting from an inflammatory process affecting the blood vessels (Wakefield et al 1989). Although this theory remains controversial, Dr Wakefield's research, featuring striking colour photographs of resin casts of sections of normal and diseased intestine, was widely praised for its originality and 'elegance'.

However, further researches in the early 1990s were not so well received. Dr Wakefield's team failed to substantiate claims that measles or measles immunisation could cause a range of inflammatory bowel conditions, and authoritative reviews have concluded that the theories cannot be sustained. Thus, even before the 1998 *Lancet* paper, Dr Wakefield was attracting controversy, although at this stage it was largely confined to specialist conferences and journals.

The publication of the *Lancet* paper and the ensuing furore accelerated the divergence between Dr Wakefield's standing in professional circles and his public popularity. Yet, rather than withdrawing his MMR–autism hypothesis, Dr Wakefield and his supporters continued to proclaim it. Having failed to convince the medical world of their hypothesis, they took the anti-MMR crusade to a wider public audience, provoking an exasperated outburst from the journal that published the original paper (see Chapter 8). Referring to Dr Wakefield's February 1998 press conference proposal that MMR be given as separate immunisations as 'a huge blow to the efforts of measles eradication', a *Lancet* editorial in May 2000 further condemned the premature disclosure of unpublished and 'uninterpretable' data by Dr Wakefield and Professor O'Leary at the congressional committee hearings in Washington in April 2000 (*Lancet* 2000). The editorial asserted that parents of autistic children 'have not been well served by these latest claims being made well beyond the publicly available evidence' and cautioned that 'a congressional hearing, like a press conference, is no place to make controversial scientific assessments'. It concluded that if scientists questioned the safety of vaccines without making their evidence fully transparent, 'harm will be done to many more children than they purport to protect' (*Lancet* 2000: 1379).

However, as Dr Wakefield's standing in the world of medicine declined, his public profile and status inexorably rose. In part, this can be attributed to the appearance of continuing divisions among medical experts over MMR, which were first exposed at the Royal Free press conference in 1998. These divisions were sustained by the high level of publicity for Dr Wakefield's allegations about the safety procedures covering the introduction of MMR in January 2001 and by a BBC Panorama programme in February 2002. The very persistence of the controversy fostered a suspicion of 'no smoke without fire' in the popular imagination, undermining confidence in the vaccine programme and causing a drop in MMR uptake.

Dr Wakefield presents an appealing image of a doctor who is informal and sympathetic, even deferential, to his patients.

'Everything I know about autism, I know from listening to parents' he earnestly confided to a Canadian interviewer (Spectrum 2000). This is a recurrent theme: in his first response to critics in *The Lancet*, he insisted that 'the approach of the clinical scientists should reflect the first and most important lesson learnt as a medical student – to listen to the patient or the patient's parent, and they will tell you the answer' (Wakefield 1998: 908). Emphasising that parents were the source of his MMR–inflammatory bowel disease–autism thesis, he claimed that this was 'a lesson in humility that, as doctors, we ignore at our peril'.

Although Dr Wakefield's self-consciously humble posture is a popular departure from the traditional image of the paternalistic doctor, it raises some questions. If it is true that he has learned everything he knows about autism from parents, this suggests that his knowledge is very limited; parents are in no position to acquire the broad scientific understanding of autism required by a medical researcher. If it is not true, which is more likely, it is merely insincere. It is also clear that the parents who brought their autistic children to see Dr Wakefield were already aware of his work suggesting a link between measles immunisation and inflammatory bowel disease. As one public health specialist commented, 'listening to the patient is important, but biased selection of patients will influence what you hear' (Walker 1998: 1355). Furthermore, Dr Wakefield appears to be highly selective in his listening: while he hears parents who endorse his views, he remains deaf to parents who do not. Nor does he appear to listen to the vast majority of his scientific and medical peers. Viewers of the Panorama documentary were shocked to discover that Dr Wakefield had not even met, never mind listened to, the parents of a child whose case was central to his argument about the 'double hit' impact of the second MMR immunisation. For all Dr Wakefield's talk about humility, his continuing public promotion of the anti-MMR cause in face of the weight of evidence to the contrary, does not suggest a surfeit of this virtue.

## Turning away from science

Dr Wakefield's appeal to the wisdom of parents and his disparagement of his scientific peers as being unduly influenced by corporate or state power, both have a deeper significance. Such notions find a ready response in a society in which currents of post-modernist relativism and cynicism run strong (Muir Gray 1999). Dr Wakefield's postures appeal to those who regard science as merely one way of understanding the natural world, and one that has an intrinsically oppressive or destructive character. The implication that, in their support for immunisation, scientists and doctors are motivated merely by greed and ambition is guaranteed a hearing at a time when the basest motives are presumed to be at the root of all individual actions. Together with the disparagement of science goes the elevation of lay wisdom and expertise. This outlook endorses the vitality and authenticity of personal experience and commonsense thinking, and asserts its superiority over experimentation and cold scientific logic. Scientists' claims to objectivity are dismissed as a mere disguise for allegiances of gender, race and class. It may seem strange, even perverse, that somebody who embarked on a career in scientific research should end up appealing to such anti-scientific prejudices, but this is one of the ironies of the MMR story.

Given the contribution of a popular anti-scientific outlook to the influence of the anti-MMR campaign, it is worth briefly clarifying the distinction between this and the scientific approach (following broadly the argument of the embryologist Lewis Wolpert in his book *The Unnatural Nature of Science*; Wolpert 1992).

### *Scientific thinking is* counter-intuitive

The laws of nature cannot be inferred from everyday experience. This is why they have remained obscure for most of human history, and why much of what science has revealed still remains obscure to most people. Science does not merely attempt to account for the unfamiliar in terms of the familiar; it often tries to explain the familiar in terms of the unfamiliar (for example, that white light can be separated into the colours of the rainbow). Wolpert emphasises how alien scientific thinking is to conventional modes of thought: 'if something fits in with commonsense, it almost certainly isn't science' (Wolpert 1992: 11).

### Commonsense *thinking serves well for everyday life, but is of little use in penetrating the mysteries of nature or the universe*

Conversely, brilliant scientists are often notoriously deficient in their dealings with the practical and the mundane. Whereas scientific thought demands self-awareness and self-criticism, rigour and consistency, commonsense does not. Folk wisdom is subjective and intuitive, based on generalising from limited experiences. Strongly influenced by emotions, folk wisdom embraces ambiguity, inconsistency and contradiction. Such modes of thought are entirely appropriate for dealing with familiar situations and social relationships. Where they fall down is in making judgements based on uncertain information, in calculating probabilities in unpredictable situations. It is therefore not surprising to find that many people experience great difficulty in making decisions that involve balancing risks, such as decisions about vaccinations.

Intuition sometimes provides clues worth pursuing in the course of clinical and scientific investigation. More often, it does not. If intuition were a reliable guide then we could all follow our feelings and hunches and science would be unnecessary. As one nineteenth-century philosopher put it, 'all science would be superfluous if the outward appearance and the essence of things directly coincided' (Marx 1894: 817). Science reveals that the evidence of our emotions, and indeed of our senses, is often misleading. For example, intuition suggests that, when one event follows another, as the diagnosis of autism does the MMR jab, then one may have caused the other. However, science tells us that association does not prove causation and scientific research has failed to reveal any link between MMR and autism.

### *Scientific knowledge is* **public** *knowledge*

Scientists develop science through interaction with other scientists and past science, by evaluating evidence and modifying their views. Their success is measured by the extent to which their theories can be shown to correspond to reality. Modern science is a collective, collaborative activity, carried out by highly selected and highly trained individuals in specialised institutions, commanding high levels of resources. Scientists cannot, like artists, work in isolation: their work is essentially cumulative and it must be validated – or falsified – by other scientists. Just as science is intrinsically subversive of tradition and authority, scientists can have no privileged sources, and ideas must be judged on their merits not on the basis of trust or deference. A set of procedures has evolved governing the organisation and commissioning of research, its publication, discussion and dissemination, as a means of ensuring that it facilitates the emergence of truth. Scientists may be no more virtuous than other citizens, but their work must conform to the evidence and must be internally consistent.

*Lorenzo's Oil,* the 1993 film starring Nick Nolte and Susan Sarandon, tells the story of how the parents of a boy – Lorenzo –

suffering from a genetically determined neurodegenerative disorder become amateur scientists and, in defiance of the medical establishment, discover a cure based on a combination of olive and rapeseed oils. Ten years later, the real Lorenzo remains profoundly handicapped and although the debate continues over whether the oil may benefit some children with this condition, it is certainly not a cure. Yet *Lorenzo's Oil* offers a myth with a powerful appeal for all parents of children with disabilities. But it is a myth. As Wolpert observes, the twentieth century provides no good example of 'the brilliant untrained scientist, working outside conventional science, perhaps in a basement, and being scorned by the Establishment' making a major scientific discovery (Wolpert 1992: 139). Dr Wakefield's assertion that 'sadly, the contribution to the understanding of autism from the medical profession and allied professions has been trivial compared to the contributions that have come from parents' is simply preposterous (and he makes no attempt to substantiate it) (Dobson 2002: 386). It remains highly improbable that any significant contribution to the understanding of autism will emerge from isolated groups of enthusiasts working in garden-shed laboratories. Meanwhile the burden such activities put on families involved is likely to be immense.

Dr Wakefield's departure to Florida, to join a research centre headed by former GP and radio talk-show host, Dr Jeff Bradstreet, completed the journey he embarked upon when he decided that listening to parents could provide the answer to scientific questions. (Dr Bradstreet is an evangelical Christian who also runs the Good News Doctor Foundation.) Dr Wakefield took another step towards abandoning science when, after failing to persuade his peers of the merits of his case, he scorned them and appealed, through sympathetic journalists, directly to members of the public who were ill-equipped to evaluate his claims. As he was feted at conferences of anti-immunisation activists and promoters of the unorthodox biomedical approach to autism, he moved even further out of the scientific mainstream. When he finally opted to continue his work in isolation, he effectively retired from serious scientific research.

One indication of Dr Wakefield's metamorphosis is the shift in his relationship to the unorthodox biomedical movement. At the outset he influenced anti-immunisation campaigners with his theories about the links between measles, MMR, inflammatory bowel disease and autism. However, as he became more estranged from the medical mainstream, the influence began to work in the opposite direction, as he incorporated themes from the wider anti-MMR campaign into his

MMR–autism hypothesis. The list of factors, in addition to MMR, that he has suggested may contribute to the emergence of autism in susceptible children is derived directly from the world of alternative health practitioners and environmental activists.

Perhaps Dr Wakefield's most appealing stance is that of the maverick against the medical establishment – the boy Andy ranged against the Goliath of the state in league with the drug companies. This has struck a particular chord at a time when there is a widespread perception of a breakdown in trust in established sources of authority, including science and medicine, doctors and politicians, capitalist corporations and the state. Dr Wakefield has assiduously promoted parallels between the MMR scare and the BSE/CJD affair. His references to 'autistic enterocolitis' as 'new variant inflammatory bowel disease' (a self-conscious parallel with 'new variant CJD') helped to make this connection. When Sir Kenneth Calman was mildly criticised in the Phillips Report (published in October 2000) for his lack of openness and urgency as Chief Medical Officer during the mad cow crisis, Dr Wakefield was quick to draw a parallel with his handling of the MMR issue.

Dr Wakefield has shown a flare for publicity in presenting his research. However, while his early public comments had a cautious and balanced character, in his subsequent statements and interviews he has become increasingly outspoken. For example, in his submission to an inquiry held by the Scottish Parliament in April 2000, he warned that 'the government's failure to wake up to the danger [of MMR] will lead to catastrophe on the scale of BSE', and implied that this was the personal responsibility of Dr Kenneth Calman, then Chief Medical Officer (Templeton 2002). He also accused his critics of being influenced by payments from vaccine manufacturers and of conducting a 'propaganda war' against him. On his departure from the Royal Free in December 2001, he was understandably bitter, claiming that his research had been delayed by 'deliberate distortion, obfuscation and political interference'. By 2002, he was displaying signs of paranoia, telling reporters that his phone was tapped, supporters were afraid of speaking openly, and that inexplicable burglaries had taken place in which cash and computers were left, but patient records were taken (Picardie 2002).

## MMR in the media

We can distinguish two phases in the media treatment of the MMR–autism link. In the three years following the appearance of

Dr Wakefield's *Lancet* paper in February 1998, the issue was largely the preserve of specialist health reporters in the broadsheet newspapers. They reported Dr Wakefield's case against MMR and the mainstream response in a balanced way. The tone was sceptical towards Dr Wakefield and tended to affirm the benefits of the mass immunisation programme. After January 2001, MMR became a major political issue: Dr Wakefield questioned the safety of the national immunisation campaign and the integrity of those running it, and the Chief Medical Officer launched a campaign of reassurance. The demand for separate vaccines gathered momentum over the next 12 months, receiving a major boost in December 2001 when Tony Blair conspicuously evaded questions about whether his son Leo had received his MMR jab. Media coverage reached a peak in February 2002 when Panorama presented a broadly sympathetic account of Dr Wakefield's case. The responsibility for covering MMR passed from reporters with expertise in scientific and medical issues to general feature writers and political correspondents. While the broadsheets now adopted a more sympathetic line towards Dr Wakefield, the tabloids, especially those hostile to the government, now jumped on the anti-MMR bandwagon.

The most prominent journalist campaigning on behalf of the anti-MMR cause is Lorraine Fraser of the *Daily Telegraph*. Under the headline 'Shame on officials who say MMR is safe' she openly endorsed Dr Wakefield's position, inaugurating a new phase of anti-MMR campaigning in the media (21 January 2001). This article is largely based on an 'exclusive interview' with Dr Wakefield who is described as 'a champion of parents who feel that their fears have been ignored'. She claims that Dr Wakefield has been 'pilloried for voicing his concerns' and that the Department of Health's 'only response to his findings has been to undermine or ignore them'. Fraser provides an uncritical account of Dr Wakefield's MMR–autism thesis and of his latest paper questioning MMR's safety. She also records Dr Wakefield's diatribe against the Department of Health for failing to recognise his work and for refusing to acquiesce to his demand for separate vaccines.

This article set the tone for a series of anti-MMR articles by Fraser (around one every month over the next two years). These reveal a close contact with Dr Wakefield and his supporters and openly endorse the anti-MMR campaign. Fraser could provide an anti-MMR spin for any story: for example, she greeted the publication of the MRC's December 2001 report (which reiterated earlier rebuttals of Dr Wakefield's case) with the headline 'Studies fail to disprove autism link to MMR jab'. (This interpretation was justified by quoting the report's caveat that it was impossible to prove the proposition that MMR never caused a case of autism, see Chapter 9). Although more experienced health correspondents remained sceptical over Dr Wakefield's claims, Fraser's partisan approach reflected a wider sympathy for his campaign and was taken up by other reporters. Indeed, so powerful had the anti-MMR consensus in the media become that Fraser was hailed as the 2002 'Health Reporter of the Year' at the British Press awards.

In May 2002, the anti-MMR campaign scored a major media coup: the publication by *Private Eye* of a 32-page MMR special (Mills 2002). Offering 'a comprehensive review of the MMR vaccination–autism controversy' – from the perspective of Dr Wakefield – this report was effectively a new campaign manifesto, superseding the document produced by the solicitor Richard Barr and colleagues in 1998 (see Chapter 7). Dr Wakefield's choice of a popular satirical magazine and a journalist with no background in science to present his case in a major scientific controversy may have seemed curious in medical and scientific circles. But it helped to confirm his maverick status and it made the case against MMR available in every newsagent's in the country.

With its presentation of the key arguments and central personalities in the campaign against MMR, the *Private Eye* special became a key source and reference for subsequent articles. Its author, Heather Mills, a journalist who, we are told, has been 'specialising in home and social affairs' for more than 20 years, provides a hagiography of Dr Wakefield as a pioneering researcher who, having discovered the cause of Crohn's disease, is now making major strides towards revealing the cause of autism. Mills quotes leading figures in the anti-MMR campaign, including the solicitor Richard Barr, Rosemary Kessick of Allergy-induced Autism and Jackie Fletcher of Jabs. Detailed accounts of a handful of children, whose parents are closely identified with the campaign, appear in this and numerous subsequent accounts. The report provides glowing endorsements of Dr Wakefield's supporters, such as Walter Spitzer, Ken Aitken and Paul Shattock. By contrast it disparages critics like Brent Taylor, Elizabeth Miller and Eric Fombonne, whose work is summarily dismissed. The counter-position of photographs of smiling campaign supporters and scowling opponents completes the report's shameless construction of pantomime heroes and villains. The report smears leading autism specialists and others involved in the MRC inquiries as 'advisors to the drug companies' – a role they only acquired as a result of the litigation against MMR. The substance of the *Private Eye* report was recycled in a series of substantial newspaper features in the following months (Cavendish 2002, Picardie 2002, Phillips 2003).

## Who duped whom?

'Public duped by media over MMR' was the headline-grabbing claim emerging from a survey published by the Economic and Social Research Council in May 2003 (Hargreaves et al 2003). According to research carried out at the Cardiff University School of Journalism, 53 per cent of those surveyed at the height of the media coverage of the MMR controversy in early 2002 believed that, because both sides of the debate received equal media coverage, there must be equal evidence for each. Although almost all scientific experts rejected the claim of a link between MMR and autism, only 23 per cent of those interviewed were aware that the bulk of evidence favoured supporters of the vaccine.

The Cardiff study, carried out by Ian Hargreaves, Justin Lewis and Tammy Speers, provides a penetrating analysis of media coverage of the MMR controversy. Compared with reports of scientific issues such as climate change and genetic research, MMR was 'most likely to be the main focus, it generated more OpEds, more letters and was given lengthier coverage on television, radio and in the press'. The authors note the generally uncritical treatment of Dr Wakefield's position, commenting that 'the connection between the MMR vaccine and autism is a speculative claim made by Wakefield with questionable scientific data to support it' (Hargreaves et al 2003: 23). Despite this, they continue, 'Wakefield's claims were not comprehensively or systematically challenged in media coverage', with the result that 'the weakness of empirical evidence in support of Wakefield's claim was never fully aired' (Hargreaves et al 2003: 23). They also note that, although there was no evidence that a single measles vaccination would be any safer than the MMR jab, the demand for separate vaccines was widely and unquestioningly taken up in the press. Although some journalists were satisfied merely to echo Dr Wakefield's views, many did try to balance their reports by indicating that the bulk of evidence supported the safety of MMR. Yet, 'attempts to balance claims about the risks of MMR jab tended merely to indicate that there were two competing bodies of evidence' (Hargreaves et al 2003: 23).

Surveys conducted by the Cardiff team revealed that, between April and October 2002, the percentage of people aware of Leo Blair's role in the story increased from 66 to 70 – 'one of the highest percentages of correct answers in both surveys'. As the authors note:

> For people confused about who to trust, this was an important indicator of the government's faith in its own position. In a nutshell, was the government's support for MMR deeply felt or merely tactical and strategic? Leo Blair might, therefore, be reasonably seen as a test of the government's confidence in its own position.
>
> (Hargreaves et al 2003: 41)

The inescapable fact that Leo's father failed this test was a serious blow to public confidence in MMR.

The media's sympathetic treatment of Dr Wakefield and the growing endorsement of the demand for separate vaccines put the government and the health authorities on the defensive. As the Cardiff study authors note, the burden of proof was placed on the side of those defending MMR (who were increasingly faced with the absurd demand to prove a negative: that MMR does *not* cause autism). The difficulties of the medical authorities were compounded when their 'dry generalisations' were met with the rhetorical force of 'emotive and sympathetic' parents who blamed MMR for making their children autistic. In a telling table, the report records that, when parents appeared as sources in newspapers, 37 were anti-MMR, 7 pro-MMR; on television, the balance was 10:3; on radio, 5:0. The authors comment that 'the use of anecdotal evidence from a selective (and unrepresentative) group of parents might also be regarded as unhelpful for such an important matter of public policy' (Hargreaves et al 2003: 44). They conclude that 'these points matter' because the media presentation of the MMR issue 'appears to have led to a loss of confidence in the vaccine in Britain', the potential public health consequences of which are 'very serious indeed' (Hargreaves et al 2003: 44).

The authors of the Cardiff study indicate that it was beyond their remit to account for the failure of journalists to question Dr Wakefield's claims. However, they acknowledge that, in the climate created by the BSE/CJD scandal, journalists were more receptive to a self-proclaimed maverick: they 'were unwilling to discount the possibility that he *may* be right' (Hargreaves et al 2003: 40). Yet, from the perspective of a school of journalism, it might be considered more alarming that so few journalists were prepared even to consider the possibility that Dr Wakefield might be wrong.

Why did the British media fall for Dr Wakefield? Perhaps, in part it was the enduring appeal of what the American mathematician Norman Levitt calls the Galileo myth – 'the idea of the lone noble genius whose insight transcends that of his hidebound age and who consequently faces scorn and persecution for his advocacy of unconventional truth' (Levitt 1999: 82). As Levitt notes, 'rarely has any cult hesitated to answer derision by resorting to this myth in some form'. Taking Dr Wakefield at his own estimation, the British press failed to realise that 'while Galileo was a rebel, not all rebels – only a tiny fraction – are Galileos' (Levitt 1999: 310). Although Galileo had some powerful sponsors, he could only have dreamed of the sort of backing that Dr Wakefield has received from the British press. Fortunately, Galileo was able to substantiate his scientific claims – something Dr Wakefield has conspicuously failed to do in the five years since he first advanced his hypothesis.

The history of science and medicine provides many examples of dissidents and heretics, of individuals who challenged conventional wisdom, suffered condemnation and rejection (or worse) only to be ultimately vindicated. The gastroenterologist Barry Marshall is a recent example. When he first suggested in 1983 that the underlying cause of the excessive acid secretion that causes peptic ulcers was a chronic infection with the bacterium Helicobacter pylori, he was met with derision. He was, after all, an Australian junior hospital doctor and his hypothesis flew in the face of conventional wisdom. Yet, within two years he had confirmed it, in part by staging a dramatic demonstration of drinking a solution of the bacterium, producing inflammation of his own stomach – confirmed by gastroscopy – and subsequently successfully treating it (LeFanu 1999: 177–86). He showed that Helicobacter was at the root of a range of diseases, including gastric and duodenal ulcers and stomach cancer, and showed that its eradication (by a simple drug regime) produced dramatic results.

Mavericks who prevail against orthodoxy have to pass two tests: they must substantiate their own hypotheses; and they must convince their peers that they are right. While Marshall spectacularly passed both tests between 1983 and 1985, since 1998, when Dr Wakefield first published his hypothesis that MMR may cause inflammatory bowel disease, which in turn may cause autism, he has conspicuously failed to pass either test.

Perhaps more significant is the fact that journalists are a key element of the professional middle-class social constituency that is at the centre of the refusal of MMR. Numerous journalists – as celebrity parents – have testified in their columns to their anxieties about MMR and, almost exclusively, to their sympathies with the anti-MMR campaign. The list includes Nigella Lawson (*The Times*), Allison Pearson (*Evening Standard*), Libby Purves (*The Times*), Suzanne Moore (*Mail on Sunday*), Lynda Lee-Potter (*Daily Mail*), Quentin Letts (*Daily Mail*), Robert Sandall (*Sunday Times*). For these columnists, writing about immunisation issues follows the principles of the 'journalism of attachment' popularised in recent military conflicts: it requires a high level of emotional engagement but no specialist knowledge of the subject. The basic qualification is having a child; a friend or relative with an autistic child is a bonus. All that is then required is a few words with Dr Wakefield and a flick through the cuttings' file.

The recent journalistic fascination with autism may also have played a part in the media's treatment of MMR. Although autism has become 'fashionable', a condition characterised by difficulties in communication remains uniquely terrifying to those who live by the word. For a profession renowned for its sociability, children for whom language and friendship are problematic are a source of potent fears.

Parents facing the decision about whether to give their children MMR, and parents of autistic children whose burden is now increased by (utterly unwarranted) fears that they may have made their children autistic by giving them MMR, have been ill-served by the media's uncritical treatment of the anti-MMR campaign. Yet it appears that the prejudice against MMR in sections of the British media is such that all critical and investigative instincts are in suspension.

## The media and MMR: three stories

### *O'Leary's apostasy*

---

*Sunday Telegraph*, 16 June 2002
REVEALED: MORE EVIDENCE TO CHALLENGE THE SAFETY OF MMR
*Government claims that vaccine presents no danger to children are undermined by tests, reports* **Lorraine Fraser**
Specialists from Trinity College, Dublin, have detected the strain of measles virus used in the MMR jab in tissue samples from the inflamed intestines of 12 children, who each developed autism after receiving the injection . . .
  Dr Wakefield said last night:

> 'Professor O'Leary and colleagues have now provided what may prove to be the most important piece of evidence to date in the case against the MMR vaccine. Parents must at the very least be given a choice of single vaccines . . .'

---

Similar stories appeared on the same day in the *Sunday Times* and the *Mail on Sunday*; another featured in the *Daily Mail* the following Monday. The articles included quotes from Dr Wakefield or a spokesman for Visceral, the charity that now supports his work. The journalists had been briefed on the contents of an unpublished paper by virologist John O'Leary, which was due to be presented at a conference in Dublin the following month. Most of the articles also referred to the fact that Dr Wakefield was due to reveal details of this work to a US congressional committee the following week.

In his statement to the Washington committee on 19 June, Dr Wakefield claimed that, 'most significantly', Professor O'Leary's work had 'confirmed that the measles vaccine virus is present in the diseased intestinal tissues of children with regressive autism'. Furthermore, 'state of the art molecular science' had shown that, in the cases of 12 children with a combination of autism and inflammatory bowel disease, the measles virus in their intestines originated in the MMR vaccine. For Wakefield these studies constituted 'a key piece of evidence in the examination of the relationship between MMR vaccine and regressive autism' (Wakefield 2002a).

However, on 16 June, in response to the articles in the British Sunday newspapers, Professor O'Leary issued a press statement that directly contradicted Dr Wakefield's interpretation of his research. Its headline stated that 'neither this publication nor any public presentation made by me or my research team has stated that MMR causes autism' (O'Leary 2002b). Referring to the work, 'which is due to be presented next month at a scientific meeting in Dublin', he insisted that 'the research in no way establishes any link between the MMR vaccine and autism'. Professor O'Leary recommended that parents give their children MMR, adding that he considered it wrong for them not to do so.

The only report of O'Leary's apostasy to appear in the British media was by Niall Dickson on the BBC television news. O'Leary's statement was subsequently quoted in a report on the British Medical Association conference on the BBC News website on 3 July 2002. None of the newspapers that reported Dr Wakefield's interpretation of Professor O'Leary's work covered O'Leary's repudiation of it.

Following Dr Wakefield's presentation in the USA, a WHO expert commented that his technique could not reliably discriminate between 'wild' and vaccine strains of measles virus. When presented with this commentary in Washington, Dr Wakefield conceded that, if this was so, 'the conclusion [of O'Leary's paper] was not justified'. Wakefield's sensational *volte face* was not reported in any British newspaper and he has yet to withdraw either his earlier claims on behalf of O'Leary or his recommendation of separate vaccines.

### Shattock's 'one in ten'

---

*Guardian*, 28 June 2002
MMR 'MAY CAUSE 1 IN 10 CASES OF AUTISM'
**James Meikle**, *Health correspondent*
The controversy over the MMR vaccine was fuelled yesterday by a researcher who suggested it might be responsible for one in ten cases of autism.

Paul Shattock, director of Sunderland University's autism research unit, believes the absence of biological markers of 'traditional' autism in the urine of some children could indicate that their condition was caused by measles.

He stressed more work was needed to establish a firm link with the triple jab, saying evidence from his unpublished study of 4,000 cases of autism was strong, but not conclusive.

---

After the news broke in an interview of Radio 4's *Today Programme* on Thursday 27 June, the story about the urine tests conducted by Mr Shattock ran through the weekend in the newspapers. Similar stories appeared on Friday in the *Daily Telegraph*, *The Times*, and the *Independent*, in the *Daily Mail*, the *Daily Express*, *The Sun* and the *Glasgow Herald*. On 30 June the *Mail on Sunday* carried references in two articles to Mr Shattock's research. On the following Monday, the *Daily Mail* featured Mr Shattock in two more articles and an editorial. These dramatic revelations were cited in support of the *Daily Mail*'s ongoing campaign for a public inquiry into the MMR–autism affair.

The 'one in ten' statistic featured prominently in all the articles. In some accounts, notably in the *Daily Mail*, the story was presented in the terrifying terms that 'one in every 1,500 MMR injections could trigger autism' (this was based on Mr Shattock's estimate that autism occurred in 1 in 150 children).

Although Mr Shattock, a pharmacist and parent of an adult autistic son, has published many articles in the 'grey literature' (in journals which have no process of evaluation or peer review), he has no record of serious scientific research. Yet he now claimed to have identified a distinct subgroup of children whose autism results from MMR: these children are said to have abnormal levels of Indolyl Acrolyl Glycine (IAG) in their urine. IAG is a breakdown product of the amino acid trytophan, which is a constituent of serotonin, melatonin and other neurotransmitters.

Although most of the above reports quoted a figure of 4,000 cases, it subsequently emerged (in a document submitted by Mr Shattock to a meeting of the Parliamentary and Science Committee on 1 July) that he had so far studied only 300 children, 10 per cent of whose parents believed that MMR caused their autism. He indicated that he did not intend to publish his results in full until he had studied 1,000 cases.

Indeed it was impossible for anybody to evaluate Mr Shattock's findings because they had not been published in any form. We do not know how his research subjects were selected, or anything about the ascertainment of diagnosis or any other aspect of the design of the study. It appears that, in these children, urinary IAG levels are abnormally low (they are apparently usually raised in autistic children). Again we know nothing about methods, controls or whether the differences were significant. Mr Shattock believes that low levels of IAG may be caused by increased gut permeability resulting from the presence of measles virus. Even if we accept that measles causes gut inflammation (which Professor O'Leary does not), it is not clear how increased gut permeability leads to low urinary IAG levels or how IAG or tryptophan are linked to autism.

Mr Shattock concedes that his studies do not prove a causal linkage between MMR and autism. However, he does believe that even these preliminary, provisional, incomplete, unvalidated and unpublished results, if taken in conjunction with the O'Leary/ Wakefield researches, indicate the need for urgent action. It is not clear whether he is calling for further research along similar lines or some action in relation to the MMR vaccine programme.

It is remarkable that any responsible newspaper should consider it legitimate to publish research findings that nobody is in a position to verify, but which are likely to have a damaging effect on the national immunisation programme and on public health. The incoherence of Mr Shattock's metabolic theory of autism should be apparent even to a journalist with no scientific training.

### The Geiers

---

*Daily Mail*, 20 May 2003
MMR RAISES RISK OF BRAIN DISORDERS, SAY RESEARCHERS
*Jenny Hope*, Medical correspondent

---

A study carried out by Mark and David Geier in the USA claimed that MMR may be a factor in up to 15 per cent of cases of autism and other neuro-developmental disorders. It was reported, first in the GP magazine *Pulse* (19 May 2003), then on the BBC News website (19 May), and in the *Daily Mail* (see above). It was thereafter widely reported on radio and television. These reports followed an earlier account of the Geiers' researches, by the veteran anti-immunisation reporter Rosie Waterhouse, in the *Daily Telegraph* on 7 April.

Mark Geier is a genetic counsellor in Maryland, USA; his son, David, is a graduate student who runs MedCon – a firm providing advice to families pursuing litigation claims over alleged vaccine injury. Although neither has any academic or professional expertise in any discipline relevant to immunisation, the Geiers feature prominently in the conferences and websites of autism activists and other anti-immunisation groups in the USA. The paper reported in the *Daily Telegraph* in April was published in the *Journal of American Physicians and Surgeons*. This sounds impressive, but turns out to be the recently relabelled *Medical Sentinel* – organ of the Association of American Physicians and Surgeons, a Right-wing medical faction based in Tucson, Arizona, distinguished by its commitment to the practice of private medicine and its hostility to immunisation. The Geier's latest paper is published in *International Pediatrics* – another apparently impressive title, this is the house journal of the Miami Children's Hospital.

In response to the paper in the *Journal of American Physicians and Surgeons*, which focused on the alleged dangers of vaccines containing the mercury-based preservative thiomersal (known as thimerosal in the USA), the American Academy of Pediatrics (AAP) published a detailed critique (AAP 2003). The most important defect of this article (shared by the *International Pediatrics* article) is its reliance on data gathered by the Vaccine Adverse Event Reporting System (VAERS). This is a passive surveillance system (analogous to the 'yellow card' reporting system in Britain) that relies on professionals and parents reporting what they suspect may be adverse reactions to vaccines. Such reports may represent true adverse events, coincidences or mistakes: 'inherent limits of VAERS include incomplete reporting, lack of verification of diagnoses, and lack of data on people who were immunised and did not report problems' (AAP 2003:1). Such data are useful for flagging up possible problems and raising questions for further investigation. They can be legitimately used for 'hypothesis generation' but not for 'hypothesis proving'.

The AAP condemned the Geiers for using data inappropriately and the paper for containing 'numerous conceptual and scientific flaws, omissions of fact, inaccuracies and misstatements'. They had 'failed to acknowledge the inherent limitations of the VAERS database when drawing conclusions of adverse event associations contained in this report and in their other publications' (AAP 2003: 1). The AAP commentary includes a 15-point catalogue of further statistical flaws, errors and omissions in the *Journal of American Physicians and Surgeons* paper.

Although their main focus is thiomersal, the Geiers are sympathetic to Dr Wakefield and his anti-MMR campaign, which has attracted considerable support in the anti-immunisation fringe in the USA. It is thus fortuitous that their researches have led to the conclusion that 'thimerosal contributed to about 75 per cent of cases of neurodevelopmental disorders, while MMR contributed to 15 per cent'. Quite apart from the methodological errors in this research and the failure of intensive previous studies to confirm these adverse effects, the notion that 90 per cent of neuro-developmental disorders can be attributed to immunisation is impossible to reconcile with the well-established genetic contribution to autism, not to mention Down's syndrome, Fragile X, tuberous sclerosis and numerous other conditions. It is extraordinary that such self-evidently preposterous claims can be taken seriously by anybody.

The Geiers' latest study plumbs new depths of absurdity (MHRA 2003). The authors compare the rates of adverse reactions following MMR (given at 15–18 months in the USA) with the rates of the same conditions reported after DTP (given at 2, 4 and 6 weeks). It is scarcely surprising to find higher rates of 'gait disturbance' in toddlers compared with infants in the first three months of life when infants are unable to walk and hence have no gait that might be disturbed. Nor is it surprising that there were more reports of autism and mental retardation among the older children: such conditions are generally not recognised until the second year of life and are certainly not likely to be identified in babies.

# 11

# EPILOGUE

## What doctors need to do

### *Put a positive case for MMR*

Doctors can do much to allay parental concerns about MMR by putting a positive case for the vaccine. Given the persistence of the MMR–autism controversy over several years and the (misleading) appearance of a major division of expert medical opinion over the safety of MMR, it is not surprising that parents are confused. Partly as a result of the involvement of some parents of autistic children in the anti-MMR campaign and their frequent appearances on television – with their children – the spectre of autism now hovers over our baby clinics. The perceived risk of autism is now more real and more immediate than that from measles, mumps and rubella – diseases of which today's parents (and even grandparents) have little memory or experience. Well-informed doctors and health visitors can help parents to make informed decisions by challenging the myth and misinformation surrounding MMR. If, when parents ask health professionals whether they had their own children immunised with MMR, they receive a positive answer, this may prove more influential than any official leaflet or poster.

The MMR scare has made it clear that a climate of anxiety and fear is not conducive to rational discussion or decision making. It is therefore important that doctors aim to reduce the emotional intensity of the MMR debate, or at least try not to provoke passions further. This means avoiding counter-scares over outbreaks of measles or the dangers of separate vaccines: these merely make parents more angry, and do not improve the uptake of MMR.

Some arguments that are pertinent at the level of immunisation policy are not necessarily the best tactics to pursue in the baby clinic.

For example, trying to make parents who are reluctant to vaccinate their children feel guilty about exposing them to the risks of measles is not likely to be effective. The accusation that they may also be exposing other people's children (some of whom may be immuno-deficient and therefore particularly vulnerable) to even greater risks may be justified, but it is more likely to provoke resentment than agreement to vaccinate. Now that the sort of consensus of support for immunisation that made requiring proof of immunisation on school entry feasible in the USA has collapsed in Britain, discussions about making immunisation compulsory here can be expected to be counter-productive. We need to rebuild a consensus for voluntary immunisation, beginning by explaining to parents why MMR is the best choice for their children.

Because of the way that MMR has become the focus of wider anxieties about environmental threats and the loss of confidence in science, medicine and government, putting the facts about immunis-ation to parents will not, in itself, be sufficient to overcome the fears and suspicions that have been stirred by the anti-MMR campaign. This requires pursuing a wider challenge to anti-vaccination propaganda and anti-science prejudices.

### *Challenging anti-vaccination propaganda*

Doctors have responded in a number of different ways to the prolif-eration of anti-vaccination propaganda over the past decade. The most common response has been to ignore it. A brief glance at the typical magazine or website reveals such a poor quality of informa-tion and argument that most doctors have concluded that the anti-vaccination movement need not be taken seriously.

However, some doctors have embraced the anti-immunisation cause. These include a few GPs, such as Jayne Donegan, expert anti-immunisation witness for the mothers refusing to immunise their children against their estranged fathers' wishes (see Chapter 3) and Peter Mansfield, who was reported to the GMC in 2001 after pub-licly promoting separate vaccines (the case was dismissed). Although few doctors have gone this far, many approve the wider accommo-dation between mainstream medicine and homeopathy, from which much anti-immunisation sentiment derives. (In a 1993 report, the British Medical Association (BMA) recommended a degree of acceptance of homeopathy, together with acupuncture, chiropractic, herbalism and osteopathy; BMA 1993.)

A third response has been opportunistic: a number of private doctors have exploited anti-immunisation fears – particularly over MMR – to make substantial profits from the provision of separate vaccines.

A combination of medical professional complacency, indulgence and opportunism has allowed the anti-vaccination movement to expand without facing any significant resistance. Within a decade its influence spread from a bohemian fringe to become a substantial force among the disaffected middle classes and beyond. Having failed to tackle this trend as it emerged from the shadows, doctors must now confront the monster it has become.

Although we can do little to stop some doctors from profiteering out of public anxieties, we can take some steps in the other two areas. We need to go to the root of the link between homeopathy and the anti-vaccination movement by clarifying the boundary between scientific medicine and non-scientific medicine. The impact of the MMR scare confirms that homeopathy is not merely a harmless fad. We should expose the absurdity of homeopathy, with its banal doctrine of similars, its dilutions beyond the laws of chemistry and its mystical tapping of potions in the Bible. We can then challenge the equally irrational anti-vaccine notions that homeopathy has promoted, such as that immunisation compromises natural immunity and may introduce susceptibility to auto-immune and other disorders in later life.

It is time that doctors, instead of turning a blind eye on anti-vaccination propaganda and allowing it to pass unchallenged, went on the offensive. The comprehensive critique that was offered by Dr Steven Conway and Professor Simon Kroll (expert witnesses for the fathers in the case of the conflicting parents) in response to the submission made by the GP/homeopath Jayne Donegan (expert witness for the mothers), greatly impressed both the trial judge, Mr Justice Sumner, and Lord Justice Sedley when the case went to the court of appeal (see Chapter 3). It is striking that, apart from being heard in court – where it was not reported – such a critique is rarely heard in public. If we are to win the case for MMR with the public, this sort of work deserves a wider readership.

Modern scientists and doctors have become remarkably diffident about standing up for the principles of science and scientific medicine. In the past, great scientists regarded the defence and advocacy of the principles of their work as an important public responsibility (Dubos 1960). They considered that it was necessary to demonstrate the superiority of their findings in debate with scientific rivals. They also considered that scientists had a responsibility to challenge popular prejudice in the process of promoting the wider enlighten-ment of society. While many of today's scientists have lost confi-dence in both themselves and society, sociologists dignify popular ignorance and prejudice as forms of lay wisdom or alternative rationality (Irwin, Wynne 1996). Raising the uptake of MMR requires a wider and more vigorous challenge to the irrational notions that have gained such an influence in modern society.

### Research into autism

Given the primitive level of our understanding of autism, the pri-ority must be to pursue basic scientific research to discover its causes and the mechanisms through which its distinctive features become manifest in human behaviour. Despite the fact that such research will not yield short-term results in terms of practical treatments, it is only through such work that effective forms of intervention will emerge in the long term.

Although autism is sometimes described as the most strongly genetically determined psychiatric disorder, extensive research has so far only confirmed the complexity of the process through which a relatively large number of genes confer a susceptibility to develop autism or a related disorder. However, the quest for such susceptibil-ity genes is important because it provides the basis for understand-ing how such genes are expressed in the neurobiological mechanisms that result in autism. It is also important in the process of trying to identify the environmental factors that contribute to the develop-ment of autism. At present notions of which environmental toxins may be relevant are derived from a familiar list, including heavy metals, certain viruses or bacteria, particular drugs or chemicals. But some agent that is generally benign may assume a pathological role in relation to a particular susceptibility gene. Thus, identifying this gene may suggest a hitherto unsuspected environmental factor.

While it is fair to say that intensive neuroscientific research has so far produced negligible therapeutic benefit, it is important to con-tinue to explore the neurobiological framework of autism. (There was a delay of around 300 years between the discovery of basic human anatomy and physiology and the emergence of effective treatments arising from this scientific framework; though this lag time has become dramatically shorter in recent years, it remains an inescapable feature of medical progress.) The study of the basic cog-nitive and emotional deficits in autism has advanced considerably, providing some guidance for strategies for influencing behaviour and learning. Again much remains to be done.

Two areas of research have been particularly neglected. The first is the evaluation of interventions, including behavioural and educational programmes and other sorts of psychological therapy or pedagogical techniques. When they are faced with a plethora of competing claims for the most diverse methods, parents need access to rigorous objective studies. The second neglected area is that of biomedical aspects of autism (which is not limited to the preoccupations of the 'unorthodox biomedical' campaigners). This includes a wide range of problems that commonly co-exist with autism, such as epilepsy, learning difficulties, anxiety and depression, obsessions and compulsions, self-injurious and aggressive behaviours, as well as gastro-intestinal disturbances.

One area that has been studied exhaustively, and in which further research would be a waste of resources, is that of speculative links with immunisations. As the American vaccine authority Paul Offitt observes, 'unfortunately, for parents who will someday bear children diagnosed with autism, the controversy surrounding vaccines has diverted attention and resources away from a number of promising leads' (Offit, 2002: 3).

### Challenging junk science

Even eminent scientists have had their careers tarnished by misinterpreting unremarkable events in a way that is so compelling that they are thereafter unable to free themselves of the conviction that they have made a great discovery. Moreover, scientists, no less than others, are inclined to see what they expect to see, and an erroneous conclusion by a respected colleague often carries other scientists along the road to ignominy. This is *pathological science*, in which scientists manage to fool themselves.

If scientists can fool themselves, how much easier is it to craft arguments deliberately intended to befuddle jurists or lawmakers with little or no scientific background? This is *junk science*. It typically consists of tortured theories of what *could be* so, with little supporting evidence to prove that it *is* so.

(Park, 2000: 9)

The relationship between mainstream and unorthodox biomedical approaches to autism parallels that between conventional medicine and anti-vaccine campaigners. The inclination of most autism experts, most of the time, is to ignore unorthodox theories and treatments. It is often only when, as happened briefly with secretin, such treatments are taken up widely by parents, that mainstream autism clinicians and researchers feel impelled to take a firm stand. Over MMR, as we have seen, most autism authorities have preferred to remain aloof from controversies in which parents have come to play a prominent role and feelings often run high. This strategy has the merit of denying more publicity to campaigners who have proved adept at manipulating public opinion. On the other hand, it carries the danger of allowing the emergence of parallel, but non-communicating, universes, one occupied by the majority of scientists and doctors, the other containing a growing body of parents, with some support from professionals. While mainstream experts confine their discussions to academic journals and conferences, parents are likely to gain access much more easily to the publications of the unorthodox trend, which are generally readily available on the Internet. The problem here is that, ultimately we, and our children, all have to live in the same world.

One alternative to ignoring the unorthodox biomedical approach is, in various ways, to adapt to it. The most extreme form of this strategy – that followed by Dr Wakefield and a small number of others – is to shift from the mainstream to the unorthodox camp and take up its outlook, in whole or in part. A more common variant is to indulge the unorthodox approach by implying a division of labour in which its advocates focus on biochemical and auto-immune aspects of autism, while mainstream scientists and clinicians deal with other aspects. This approach has become commonplace at conferences run by parent groups at which speakers from both trends present their work. This inclusive strategy allows for some discussion between representatives of different trends, and fosters a degree of unity, however uneasy, within the world of autism. The danger of this approach is that, when advocates of unorthodox approaches appear on the same platforms as mainstream experts, it gives a degree of legitimacy to their work that it might otherwise lack (this may explain why they are enthusiastic participants in such events).

There is a remarkable reluctance of established autism authorities either to publicise work that indicates the deficiencies of particular unorthodox biomedical approaches or to respond critically to the misuse of mainstream research by unorthodox campaigners. For example, parents are still sending their children's urine specimens for testing in private laboratories in Britain and the USA, and full details of these tests and their alleged significance is available over the Internet. Yet an excellent study carried out in Edinburgh that confirms the uselessness of these tests is buried in an academic journal where it is unknown and inaccessible to parents (Hunter, O'Hare 2003). To take another example, in a paper supporting Dr Wakefield's MMR–autism thesis, Dr Kenneth Aitken quotes the results of a pilot study of a screening test for autism as though this provides authoritative figures for diagnosis of autism (Aitken 1999). Although I have heard members of the team privately denounce this abuse of their research, I have been unable to find any public statement to this effect. Meanwhile, Dr Aitken's paper has been freely available on the Internet since 1999.

The convergence of anti-vaccination and unorthodox biomedical activists in the campaign against MMR, and the significant public impact they have achieved, confirm the urgency of making a clearer distinction between serious and junk science in the world of autism. The price paid for inclusiveness is a loss of coherence, which is likely to make life even more difficult for children with autism and their families. If serious scientists have done work, which shows that the tests and treatments that some parents are pursuing for their children are unreliable and ineffective, this should be made available to them in an accessible form. Rather than fudging the differences between mainstream science and unorthodox approaches, scientists should help parents to distinguish between interventions that may be beneficial and those that are not, by subjecting unorthodox theories to a comprehensive critique.

## What we need to do together

My job is to love him; your job is to keep him well.
(Mitchell 2000: 1)

What Lesli Mitchell calls her 'implicit contract' with her doctor over her autistic son might well be extended to the scientists and other professionals engaged in the diverse fields of autism research and intervention: 'your job is to find out what is wrong with him and work out the most effective ways of treating him'. Parents and doctors and other professionals share a common commitment to the advance of the scientific study of autism, but their perspective is different. One of the problems arising from the new wave of parent activism in autism is a shift away from the division of labour implied in Lesli Mitchell's contract and a significant blurring of the boundaries between parents and professionals.

In recent years, parents have increasingly taken on a range of what were formerly regarded as professional roles. Some parents have become therapists in home educational programmes, or teachers in special schools set up by parents faced with a lack of state provision. Others have taken on at least some of the responsibilities of scientists or doctors, intensively researching the subject and administering experimental dietary or other treatments to their children. Others have become expert litigants, campaigners, lobbyists and fundraisers. Although some parents have successfully pursued several of these courses, the majority of parents are, not least because of the pressures of having an autistic child, unable to pursue any of them. And even for the parents who are most successful, there is an inescapable tension between these additional roles and their primary role as parent (not to mention the often-associated roles as parent of other, non-autistic, children, partner, member of wider family, wage or salary earner). The breakdown in the division of labour between parents and professionals means that some parents are shouldering an unsustainable burden that inevitably impinges on their role as parents.

In part, the plight of parents of autistic children must be set in the context of wider political forces acting on patients and parents. In response to the perception of growing disengagement from the political process, politicians have sought to compensate for the loss of legitimacy resulting from the 'democratic deficit' by extending public participation in areas such as health (in which the rapid growth of disease-related voluntary organisations and charities reflects a high level of popular involvement). Authorities in science and medicine, perceiving (and, perhaps, exaggerating) a loss of public trust in their activities, have welcomed moves towards tighter official regulation and greater public involvement in their activities. Sensing the insecurity of the medical and allied professions, politicians have discovered that denunciations of traditional 'paternalism' have a popular resonance and ensure a feeble and defensive response from professionals to modernising initiatives. For example, the 'expert patient' initiative, launched by the Department of Health in 2001, implied that some patients knew more about their conditions than their doctors and sought to extend this expertise through local programmes (DH 2001: 5). Influential health and social policy think-tanks have promoted this agenda of patient autonomy against traditional paternalism (Coulter 2002, Harrison, New 2002).

Instead of trying to restore democracy to the political process, where it is sorely lacking, politicians are now purporting to extend it to the spheres of science and medicine, where it is inappropriate. Science is an inherently hierarchical activity: its practitioners are selected on the basis of their superior aptitude in a particular sphere and appointed to professorial or other high office (at least in principle) according to their record of scientific achievement. In the world of politics, the concept 'one person – one vote' reflects a fundamental egalitarian principle. In science, however, people are not equal and success depends on recruitment and advancement on the basis of ability and merit. Those at the top of scientific hierarchies should be accountable to public authorities, particularly when they are receiving public funding, and should be required to justify the judgements on research priorities that they have made on scientific grounds. But the day-to-day processes of scientific research, from the award of research grants to the design and conduct of programmes, cannot be conducted according to democratic principles.

Given the significance of science in society and the level of public interest in it, it is important that scientific agencies attempt to explain their work to the public. But this is not the same as inviting public participation in deciding on the content or direction of scientific research. In practice, there is little that is democratic about the new forms of public involvement in science and medicine, which generally involve the appointment of prominent members of campaigning groups to particular committees. These individuals are not representative (indeed they are inevitably highly unrepresentative) and they are in no way accountable to the collective of patients or parents of which they are members. They are inherently susceptible to being patronised or manipulated by the professional authorities (unless they represent substantial fundraising potential, in which case the manipulation may well operate in the opposite direction). In the former case, the patients or parents suffer, as token consultation processes legitimise decisions taken elsewhere; in the latter, the science is likely to suffer, as research projects that might not satisfy more scientifically informed scrutiny win approval.

Another wider trend – well exemplified in the notion of the 'expert patient' – is the denigration of scientific and professional expertise. This is apparent in relation to the two areas we have considered in this book: autism and immunisation. In both areas there is a vast scientific literature and substantial areas of overlap with other disciplines, such as psychology, paediatrics, immunology and infectious diseases. A scientist or doctor working in either field requires a familiarity with the basic medical sciences, together with postgraduate specialisation: this means at least ten years of study and training. Few parents of autistic children, or parents faced with decisions about immunisation, are in a position to become 'expert patients', if only because of limitations of time and energy. Campaigners against medical paternalism believe that it is patronising to parents to suggest that doctors or scientists may know more about their children's condition than they do. But this is absurd. The truth is that it is disparaging to science and medicine to suggest that expert knowledge and skills can be so readily acquired.

The rejection of medical paternalism has a populist appeal. But the radical aura of this sceptical attitude towards established sources of scientific and medical authority is tarnished by the fact that it is often accompanied by credulity towards alternative sources of authority, such as anti-vaccination campaigners whose claims lack any scientific validity and cannot stand up to critical scrutiny. In contemporary society, scepticism about scientific authority often expresses a corrosive cynicism about the possibility of any objective knowledge of the world and a repudiation of any concept of human agency.

Critics of medical paternalism argue that doctors should simply provide patients with 'the full facts' and allow them to make their own decisions about matters such as immunisations (Coulter 2002: 118). Quite apart from the problem that 'the full facts' in any such controversy are highly contested, this argument overestimates the value of information and underestimates the problem of interpreting the mass of information that is all too readily available. When scientists are confronted with results from an unfamiliar area of research, they do not customarily try to close down the areas of uncertainty by seeking further information from alternative sources. For example, in his account of the MMR controversy, Professor John Walker-Smith, senior paediatric gastroenterologist in the Wakefield team, indicates his problem in evaluating the results of Professor John O'Leary's specialised molecular techniques, about which conflicting claims have been made:

> Such a situation poses a difficulty for a clinician where one does not have personal technical expertise, one has to make a human judgement based up on the quality of the person doing the work and his reputation. For me I have complete

faith in the integrity of his findings and the quality of the work coming from John O'Leary's laboratory.

(Walker-Smith 2003: 245-6)

In other words, the basis on which one scientist puts faith, at least provisionally, in another's findings is not information, but trust. Professor Walker-Smith further emphasises that 'scientific rigour demands these must be confirmed independently in another laboratory' (which, so far, they have not).

Just as trust is the crucial factor in relationships between scientists, so it is in relationships between doctors and scientists on the one hand, and patients and parents on the other (Brewin 1985, O'Neill 2002). The weakening of trust in these relationships has led patients and parents to seek to acquire scientific and medical expertise – a trend encouraged for their own purposes by politicians and the medical establishment. But, for the vast majority of patients, even if they have advanced medical or scientific qualifications, it is imposs-ible to overcome the gulf in knowledge and expertise between them and a specialist in autism or immunisation. The attempt to do so can only intensify distrust in professionals, while imposing an intolerable burden on already overstretched parents. Instead of trying to close the information gap, we need to find ways of rebuilding trust.

We need to establish the foundations of an informal contract between parents and professionals that respects both our different spheres of expertise and – most importantly – the distinctions between them. Whether we are parents concerned about immunisa-tion or parents of autistic children, doing the best for our children means concentrating on being parents and leaving science to the scientists, medicine to the doctors, education to the teachers. So influential has the rhetoric of anti-paternalism become that this now appears a hopelessly old-fashioned proposal. But it is both prin-cipled and pragmatic. If I am having trouble with my car, I do not take to the Internet to study motor engineering; I take it to a garage and ask the mechanic to repair it. Even though I do not understand his explanation of the problem and I worry about how much it is going to cost, I trust him. In a similar way, we put our trust in numerous people we encounter in our everyday lives. If we did not, society would simply collapse. The peculiarity of our current predica-ment is the selective withdrawal of trust from scientific and medical professionals, which is both unjustified and mutually damaging.

As parents, we look to medical and scientific experts to provide some answers to our questions about autism. We expect doctors to listen to us, but we also expect them to bring to bear the results of examination and investigation, clinical experience and research, a whole body of knowledge and expertise. We expect more of scientists involved in research as well as clinical practice. We expect them to stand back from our highly subjective and emotionally burdened engagement with the problems of autism to pursue objective, dispassionate inquiries.

We need scientists to pursue research of the highest quality, according to the standards of science, not those of the mass media. We should expect them not to raise parents' hopes, or fears, prematurely, with provisional, unvalidated results. We should expect them to present their results, in the first instance, to fellow scientists, in the private sphere of expert conferences and professional journals, not in the public world of conferences involving parents, the popular press and the Internet. If the proper process of scientific discussion leads to the confirmation of some new theory or treatment, then its authors are entitled to present their work to a wider audience (even if their innovation is not universally approved by colleagues). But if scientists turn to the mass media in response to their failure to convince a substantial body of their peers of the validity of their work, this is likely to be bad for science and confusing to the public (and it may be, as in the case of MMR, damaging to public health). (In these circumstances, we might also expect a responsible press to exercise restraint in publicising such work.)

Scientists in turn are entitled to be allowed to get on with their work without excessive public interference. If more high-quality scientific research secured substantial institutional funding, there would be less pressure on researchers to resort to the mass media and appeals to parent organisations to finance their work. If parents or patients decide to take an interest in scientific research, they should be patient and realistic: it is unreasonable to expect that any current research will lead to practical applications in the short term.

The MMR–autism controversy reveals the dangers of the growth of irrationality in society. As a result of a complex combination of factors, irrational anti-immunisation sentiments and irrational theories about autism have gained widespread popularity, potentially undermining the effectiveness of the national child immunisation programme. Unless we begin to confront this wave of irrationality, the consequences could be grave, and they will not be confined to the sphere of health. As Stevie Wonder puts it:

# EPILOGUE

When you believe in things that you don't understand,
Then you suffer,
Superstition ain't the way.

(Wonder 1972)

# BIBLIOGRAPHY

*Note: Internet sites accessed between January and December 2003.*

Abbasi, K. (2001) 'Man, mission, rumpus', *British Medical Journal*; 322: 306.

Afzal, M.A., Minor, P.D., Begley, J., Bentley, M.L, Armitage, E., Ghosh, S., Ferguson, A. (1998a) 'Absence of measles-virus genome in inflammatory bowel disease', *Lancet*; 351: 646–7.

Afzal, M.A., Armitage. E., Begley, J. et al. (1998b) 'Absence of detectable measles virus genome sequence in IBD tissues and peripheral blood lymphocytes', *Journal of Medical Virology*; 55: 293–9.

Afzal, M.A., Osterhaus, A.D.M.E., Cosby, S.L., Jin, L., Beeler, J., Takeuchi, K., Kawashima, H. (2003) 'Comparative evaluation of measles virus-specific RT-PCR methods through an international collaborative study', *Journal of Medical Virology*; 70: 171–6.

Aitken, K.J. (2001a) 'Expert Group Presentation', Health and Community Care Committee, Scottish Assembly at www.show.scot.nhs.uk/mmrexpert group/Aitken-rep.htm.

Aitken, K.J. (2001b) 'Q&A' at www.singlevaccines.com/ken-aitken1.html.

Alexander Harris (2000) See www.alexharris.co.uk/mpa_mmr.asp.

Allergy Induced Autism (1999) Statement on Taylor et al 1999, at www.whale.to/vaccines/aia.html.

American Academy of Pediatrics (2003) 'Study fails to show a connection between thimerosal and autism', www.aap.org/profed/thimaut-may03.htm.

Anon (2000) 'MMR vaccine and autism', Editorial, *Adverse Drug Reactions and Toxicological Review*; 19 (2): 99–100.

Anon (2003) 'MMR vaccine – how effective and how safe?', *Drug and Therapeutics Bulletin*; 41 (4): 25–9.

Arlett, P., Bryan, P. (2001) 'A response to "MMR: through a glass, darkly" by Drs AJ Wakefield and SM Montgomery and published reviewers' comments', *Adverse Drug Reactions and Toxicological Review*; 20 (1): 37–45.

Asperger, H. (1961) 'Die Psychopathologie des coeliakiekranken Kindes', Coeliake-Symposium. Belp BE, *Ann. Paediat;* 197: 346–51.

Asperger, H. (1991) '"Autistic psychopathology" in childhood', (originally published in 1944 in German, translated and annotated by Uta Frith), in U. Frith (ed) *Autism and Asperger Syndrome*, pp 37–92, Cambridge: Cambridge University Press.

Badenoch, J. (1988) 'Big bang for vaccination' (Editorial), *British Medical Journal*; 297: 750–1.

Bailey, A., Le Couteur, A., Gottesman, I., Bolton, P., Simonoff, E., Yuzda,E. (1995) 'Autism as a strongly genetic disorder: evidence from a British twin study', *Psychological Medicine*; 25 (1): 63–77.

Baird, G., Charman, T., Baron-Cohen, S., Cox, A., Swettenham, J., Wheelwright, S., Drew, A. (2000) 'A screening instrument for autism at 18 months of age: a six year follow-up study', *Journal of the American Academy of Child and Adolescent Psychiatry*; 39: 694–702.

Baker, J.P. (2003) 'The pertussis vaccine controversy in Great Britain, 1974–1986', *Vaccine*; 21: 4003–10.

Bandolier (2002) 'MMR vaccination' at www.jr2.ox.ac.uk/bandolier/band84/MMR.html

Baron Cohen, S. (1995) *Mindblindness: An essay on autism and theory of mind*, Boston: MIT press/Bradford Books.

Baron Cohen, S., Wheelwright, S., Cox, A., Baird, G., Charman, T., Swettenham, J., Drew, A., Doehring, P. (2000) 'Early identification of autism by the Checklist for Autism in Toddlers (CHAT)', *Journal of the Royal Society of Medicine*; 93: 521–5.

Barr, R., Limb, K. (1998) *Measles, mumps, rubella vaccines (MMR or MR): information pack*, London: Hodge, Jones and Allen (solicitors), now available at www.alexharris.co.uk.

Bedford, H., Elliman, D. (2001) *Childhood Immunisation: The facts*, London: Health Promotion England.

Bettelheim, B. (1967) *The Empty Fortress: Infantile autism and the birth of the self*, New York: Free Press.

BMA (British Medical Association) (1993) *Complementary Medicine: New approaches to good practice*, London: BMA.

BMA (2003) *Childhood Immunisation: A guide for healthcare professionals*, BMA Board of Science and Education, London: BMA.

Bolton, P.F., Rutter, M. (2001) 'Genetic influences in autism', *International Review of Psychiatry*; 2: 67–80.

Bowie, C. (1990) 'Lessons from the pertussis vaccine trial', *Lancet*, 335: 397–9.

Brewin, T. (1985) 'Truth, trust and paternalism', *Lancet* (31 August): 490–2.

Bristol-Power, M. (2001) 'The Etiology of Autism and National Institute of Child Health and Human Development Research', presentation to the Institute of Medicine Safety Review Committee, held at the National Academy of Sciences, Washington, DC, at www.nichd.gov/autism/IOM_presentation.htm.

Brown, D.W.G., Jin, L., Ramsay, M. (2002) 'Comments on abstract summission', *Infectious Diseases in the News* (27 June), London: Public Health Laboratory Service (www.phls.org.uk/press).

Brynner, R., Stephens, T. (2001) *The Impact of Thalidomide and its Revival as a Vital Medicine*, Cambridge, MA: Perseus.

Buie, T., Winter, H., Kushak, R. (2002) 'Preliminary findings in gastro-intestinal investigation of autistic patients', at www.autismnwaf.com/harvardproject2.htm.

Butler, D., Kavanagh, D. (eds) (2001) *The British General Election of 2001*, London: Palgrave Macmillan.

Calman, K. (1998) 'MMR vaccine, Crohn's disease and autism', *From the Chief Medical Officer*, (27 March).

Caplin, C. (2004) 'Why is no one allowed to question MMR?', *Night & Day (Mail on Sunday)*, 29 February.

Chadwick, N., Bruce, I.J, Schepelmann, S., Pounder, P.E., Wakefield, A.J. (1998) 'Measles virus RNA is not detected in IBD using hybrid capture and reverse transcription followed by PCR', *Journal of Medical Virology*; 55: 305–11.

Chaitow, L. (1987) *Vaccination and Immunisation: Dangers, delusions and alternatives (what every parent should know)*, Saffron Walden: Daniel.

Chen, R.T., DeStefano, F. (1998) 'Vaccine adverse events: causal or coincidental?', *Lancet*, 351: 611–12.

Chez, M., Buchanan, C.T., Bagan, B.T., (2000) 'Secretin and autism: a two-part clinical investigation', *Journal of Autism and Developmental Disorders*; 30: 87–94.

Clark, W.R. (1995) *At War Within: The double-edged sword of immunity*, Oxford: Oxford University Press.

Coleman, M. (1997) 'Autism and coeliac disease', in G. Gobbi et al (eds) *Epilepsy and Other Neurological Disorders in Coeliac Disease*, pp 219–21, London: Libbey.

Collier, J.A.B., Longmore, J.M., Hodgetts, T.J. (1997) *Oxford Handbook of Clinical Specialities*, fourth edn, Oxford: Oxford University Press.

Committee on Safety of Medicines (1995) 'Adverse reactions to measles rubella vaccine', *Current Problems in Pharmacovigilance*; 21: 9–10.

Communicable Disease Surveillance Centre (1995) 'The national measles and rubella campaign – one year on', *CDR Weekly*; 5 (45): 237.

Connell, P.H. (1966) 'Medical treatment', in J.K. Wing (ed), *Early Childhood Autism: Clinical, educational and social aspects*, Oxford: Pergamon.

Coulter, A. (2002) *The Autonomous Patient: Ending paternalism in medical care*, London: Nuffield Trust/Stationery Office.

Coulter, H.L., Fisher, B.L. (1985) *DPT: Shot in the dark*, (1991 edn), Avery Publishing Group.

Croen, L.A., Grether, J.K., Hoogstrate, J., Selvin, S. (2002) 'The changing prevalence of autism in California', *Journal of Autism and Developmental Disorders*, 32 (3): 207–15.

Dales, L., Hammer, S., Smith, N. (2001) 'Time trends in autism and in MMR immunisation coverage in California', *Journal of the American Medical Association*; 285 (9): 1183–85.

Davis, R.L. et al (2001) 'MMR and other measles-containing vaccines do not increase the risk for inflammatory bowel disease', *Archives of Pediatric and Adolescent Medicine*; 155: 354–9.

Dealler, S. (1999) 'A chemical aetiology for autism spectrum disorders: opioid peptides and secretin', paper submitted to Autism 99 internet conference at trainland.tripod.com/stephen.htm.

Dealler, S. (2001) 'MMR and toxicology', *Adverse Drug Reactions and Toxicology Review*; 20 (1): 55–7.

Deer, B. (1998) 'But what if the law got it wrong?', *Sunday Times Magazine*, 1 November (see 'The vanishing victims', briandeer.com/dtp-dpt-vaccine. htm.)

Deer, B. (2004a) 'The truth behind the crisis', *Sunday Times*, 22 February.

Deer, B. (2004b) 'Key ally of MMR doctor rejects autism link', *Sunday Times*, 7 March.

D'Eufemia, P., Celli, M., Finocchiaro, R. (1996) 'Abnormal intestinal permeability in children with autism', *Acta Paediatrica*, 85: 1076–9.

DeWilde, S., Carey, I.M., Richards, S., Hilton, S.R., Cook, D.G. (2001) 'Do children who become autistic consult more often after MMR vaccination?', *British Journal of General Practice*; 51: 226–7.

DH (Department of Health) (1997) *On the State of the Public Health: The annual report of the Chief Medical Officer of the Department of Health for the year 1996*, London: HMSO.

DH (2001) *Expert Patients*, (Report of Expert Patients Task Force), London: DH.

DH (2002a) *Report of the CFS/ME Working Group*, London: DH.

DH (2002b) *MMR: Information for parents*, June, London: DH (see also www.mmrthefacts.nhs.uk).

DH (2002c) 'Critique on recent Singh paper', August, www.mmrthefacts. nhs.uk/news/newsitem.php?id=34&start=1.

Dineen, T. (1999) *Manufacturing Victims: What the psychology industry is doing to people*, London: Constable.

Dobson, R. (2002) 'Parents' champion or loose cannon', *British Medical Journal*; 324: 386.

Donald, A., Muthu, V. (2002) 'No evidence that MMR vaccine is associated with autism or bowel disease', *Clinical Evidence*, 7: 331–40.

Dubos, R. (1960) *Louis Pasteur: Freelance of science*, New York: Da Capo.

Dyer, C. (1994) 'Families win support for vaccine compensation claim', *British Medical Journal*; 309: 759.

Dyer, O. (2002) 'Experts question latest MMR research', *British Medical Journal*; 325: 354.

Egan, S., Logan, G., Bedford, H. (1994) 'Low uptake of immunisation; associated factors and the role of health education initiatives' in Health Education Authority (ed) *Uptake of Immunisation: Issues for health education*, London: Health Education Authority.

Elliman, D., Bedford, H. (2001) 'MMR vaccine: the continuing saga', *British Medical Journal*; 322: 183–4.

Farrington, C.P., Miller, E., Taylor, B. (2001) 'MMR and autism: further evidence against a causal association', *Vaccine*; 19: 3632–5.

Fernandez-Armesto, F. (2001) *Food: A history*, London: Pan.

Feudtner, C., Marcuse, E.K. (2001) 'Ethics and immunization policy: promoting dialogue to sustain consensus', *Pediatrics*; 107 (5): 1158–64.

Finn, A. (2002) 'MMR vaccine debate: competing interests need to be declared' (Letter), *British Medical Journal*; 324: 734–5.

Fitzpatrick, M. (1998) 'How now mad cow?' in I. McCalman with B. Penny and M. Cook (eds), *Mad Cows and Modernity: Cross disciplinary reflections on the crisis of Creutzfeldt-Jakob Disease*, Humanities Research Centre Monograph Series No. 13, Canberra: Australian National University.

Fitzpatrick, M. (2001) *The Tyranny of Health: Doctors and the regulation of lifestyle*, London: Routledge.

Fitzpatrick, M. (2002a) 'Myalgic Encephalomyelitis: the dangers of Cartesian dualism', *British Journal of General Practice*; 52: 432–3.

Fitzpatrick, M. (2002b) 'The surrender of scientific medicine', in *Alternative Medicine: Should we swallow it?*, London: Institute of Ideas/Hodder and Stoughton.

Fletcher, A.P. (2000) 'Referee 3' (comments on 'MMR vaccine: through a glass darkly' by A.J. Wakefield and S.M. Montgomery) *Adverse Drug Reactions and Toxicology Reviews*; 19 (4): 288–91.

Fombonne, E. (1998) 'Inflammatory bowel disease and autism', (Research letters), *Lancet*: 352: 955.

Fombonne, E. (2001) 'Is there an epidemic of autism?', *Pediatrics*; 411–3.

Fombonne, E. (2002) 'Prevalence of childhood disintegrative disorder', *Autism*; 6 (2) 149–57.

Fombonne, E., Chakrabarti, S. (2001) 'No evidence for a new variant of MMR-induced autism', *Paediatrics*, 108 (4) at pediatrics.org/cgi/content/full/108/4/e58.

Frith, U. (1989) *Autism: Explaining the enigma*, Oxford: Blackwell.

Frith, U. (ed) (1991) *Autism and Asperger Syndrome*, Cambridge: Cambridge University Press.

Fudenberg, H.H. (undated) 'Specific therapies for different disorders within the autistic spectrum' , www.nitrf.org.

Fudenberg, H.H. (1996) 'Dialysable lymphocytic extract (DlyE) in infantile onset autism: a pilot study', *Biotherapy*; 9 (1–3): 143–7.

Furedi, F. (2002) *Culture of Fear: Risk-taking and the morality of low expectations*, revised edn, London/New York: Continuum.

Furlano, R.I., Anthony, A., Day, R., Brown, A., McGarvey, L., Thomson, M.A., Davies, S.E., Berelowitz, M., Forbes, A., Wakefield, A.J., Walker-Smith, J.A., Murch, S.H. (2001) 'Colonic CD8 and gammadelta-cell infiltration with epithelial damage in children with autism', *Journal of Pediatrics*; 138: 366–72.

Galambos, L. (1999) 'A century of innovation in vaccines', *Vaccine*; 17: S7–10.

Gallagher, R. (2003) 'Vaccination undermined', *The Scientist*; 17 (22) (17 November): 6.

Gangarosa, E.J., Galazka, A.M., Wolfe, C.R., Phillips, L.M., Gangarosa, R.E., Miller, E., Chen, R.T. (1998) 'Impact of anti-vaccine movements on pertussis control: the untold story', *Lancet*, 351: 356–61.

Gay, N.J., Miller, E. (1995) 'Was a measles epidemic imminent?', *Communicable Disease Report*; 5 (13): R204–7.

Gay, N., Ramsay, M., Cohen, B., Hesketh, P., Morgan-Capner, P., Brown, D. Miller, E. (1997) 'The epidemiology of measles in England and Wales since the 1994 vaccination campaign', *Communicable Disease Report*; 7 (2): R17–21.

Geier, M.R., Geier, D.A. (2003a) 'Thimerosal in childhood vaccines, neuro-developmental disorders and heart disease in the United States', *Journal of American Physicians and Surgeons*, 8: 6–11.

Geier, M.R., Geier, D.A. (2003b) 'Pediatric MMR vaccination safety', *International Pediatrics*, 18 (2): 108–13

Gershon, M.D. (2001) 'Testimony to the Congress of the United States House of Representatives Committee on Government Reform: hearing on "The challenges of autism: why the increased rates?"' (April) at www.house.gov/reform/hearings/healthcare/01.04.25/gershon.htm.

Gevitz, N. (1993) 'Unorthodox medical theories' in W.F. Bynum and R. Porter (eds) *Companion Encyclopedia of the History of Medicine*, London: Routledge.

Gillberg, C., Coleman, M. (2000) *The Biology of the Autistic Syndromes*, Cambridge: Cambridge University Press.

Gillberg, C., Heijbel, H. (1998) 'MMR and autism', *Autism*, 2 (4): 423–4.

Gillberg, C., Wing, L. (1999) 'Autism: not an extremely rare disorder', *Acta Psychiatrica Scandinavica*; 99: 399–406.

Gillberg, C., Steffenburg, S., Schaumann, H. (1991) 'Is autism more common now than ten years ago?', *British Journal of Psychiatry*; 158: 403–9.

Golden, G.S. (1990) 'Pertussis vaccine and injury to the brain', *Journal of Pediatrics*; 116: 854–61.

Government Statistical Service (2003) *National Immunisation Statistics, England: 2001–02,* London: Government Statistical Service.

Greenhalgh, T. (2001) *How to Read a Paper: The basics of evidence-based medicine*, second edn, London: BMJ.

Gupta, S. (2000) 'Immunological treatments for autism', *Journal of Autism and Developmental Disorders*; 30 (5) (October): 475–9.

Gupta, S., Aggarwal, S., Heads, C. (1996) 'Dysregulated immune system in children with autism: beneficial effects of intravenous immunoglobulin on autistic characteristics', *Journal of Autism and Developmental Disorders*; 26 (4) (August): 439–52.

Hall, G. (2000) 'The MMR litigation – where next? How soon?': causation issues to be resolved by invasive tests on infants', *Medical Litigation*, October.

Halsey, N.A. et al (2001) 'MMR vaccine and autistic spectrum disorder: a report from the new challenges in childhood immunisation conference', *Pediatrics*; 107 (5): e84.

Hargreaves, I., Lewis,J., Speers,T. (2003) 'Towards a better map: science, the public and the media', London: Economic and Social Research Council.

Harrison, A., New, B. (2002) *Public Interest, Private Decisions: Health-related research in the UK*, London: King's Fund.

Healy, D. (2002) *The Creation of Psychopharmacology*, Cambridge, MA: Harvard University Press.

Hess, D. (1997) *Can Bacteria Cause Cancer? Alternative medicine confronts big science*, New York/London: New York University Press.

Hobson, P. (2002) *The Cradle of Thought: Exploring the origins of thinking*, London: Palgrave Macmillan.

Hocking, B. (1987) *The Independent*, 3 November.

Horton, R. (2003) *Second Opinion: Doctors, diseases and decisions in modern medicine*, London: Granta.

Horvath, K., Stefanatos, G., Sokolowski, K.N., Wachtel, R., Nabors, L., Tildon, J.T. (1998) 'Improved social and language skills after secretin in patients with autism spectrum disorders', *Journal of the Association of Academic Minority Physicians*; 9: 9–15.

Horvath, K., Papadimitriou, M.D., Rabsztyn, A., Drachenberg, C., Tildon, J.T. (1999) 'Gastrointestinal abnormalities in children with autistic disorder', *Journal of Pediatrics*; 135: 559–63.

Houston, R., Frith, U. (2000) *Autism in History: The case of Hugh Blair of Borgue*, Oxford: Blackwell.

Howlin, P. (1998) 'Practitioner review: psychological and educational treatments for autism', *Journal of Child Psychology and Psychiatry and Allied Disciplines*, 39: 307–22.

Hunter, L.C., O'Hare, A., Herron, W.J., Fisher, L.A., Jones, G.E. (2003) 'Opioid peptides and dipeptidyl peptidase in autism', *Developmental Medicine and Child Neurology*; 45: 121–8.

Institute of Medicine (2001) *Immunisation Safety Review: Measles-Mumps-Rubella vaccine and autism*, Washington, DC: National Academy of Sciences.

Institute of Medicine (2003) *Financing Vaccines in the 21st Century: Assuring access and availability*, Washington, DC: Institute of Medicine.

Irwin, A., Wynne, B. (eds) (1996) *Misunderstanding Science? The public reconstruction of science and technology*, Cambridge: Cambridge University Press.

Jick, H., Kaye, J.A. (2003) 'Epidemiology and possible causes of autism', *Pharmacotherapy*; 23 (12): 1524–30.

Joliffe, T., Lansdowne, R., Robinson, C (1992) 'Autism: a personal account', *Communication*, 26 (3), December.

Jordan, R. (1999) *Autistic Spectrum Disorders: An introductory handbook for practitioners*, London: David Fulton.

Jordan, R., Jones, G. (1999) *Meeting the Needs of Children with Autism Spectrum Disorders*, London: David Fulton.

Jordan, R., Jones, G., Murray, D. (1998) *Educational Interventions for Children with Autism: A literature review of recent and current research*, Research Report 77, London: Department for Education and Employment.

Kallen, R.J. (1999a) 'Secretin: a treatment for autism', Autism Biomedical Information Network, www.autism-biomed.org/secretin.htm.

Kallen, R.J. (1999b) 'What about "it can't hurt to try" a new treatment?', Autism Biomedical Information Network, www.autism-biomed.org/canthurt.htm.

Kallen, R.J. (2000) 'Unproven treatments', Autism Biomedical Information Network, www.autism-biomed.org/unproven.htm.

Kanner, L. (1943) 'Autistic disturbances of affective contact', *Nervous Child*; 2: 217–50.

Kaye, J.A., Melero-Montes, M., Jick, H. (2001) 'MMR vaccine and the incidence of autism recorded by GPs: a time-trend analysis', *British Medical Journal*; 322: 460–3.

Kidd, I,M., Booth, C, J., Rigden, S.P.A., Tong, C.Y.W, MacMahon, E.M.E. (2003) 'Measles-associated encephalitis in children with renal transplants: a predictable effect of waning herd immunity?' *Lancet*; 362: 832.

Killick Millard, C. (1948) 'The end of compulsory vaccination', *British Medical Journal*, (18 December): 1074.

King, S. (1999) 'Vaccination policies: individual rights *v* community health', *British Medical Journal*; 319: 1448–9.

Knivsberg, A.M., Reichelt, K.L., Nodland, M., Holen, T. (1995) 'Autistic syndromes and diet: a four year follow-up study', *Scandinavian Journal of Educational Research*; 39: 223–36.

Krigsman, A. (2002) 'Testimony before the Committee on Government Reform', 'The status of research into vaccine safety and autism'. Washington DC: Congressional Committee on Government Reform; www.house.gov/search.

Kroll-Smith, S., Hugh Floyd, H. (1997) *Bodies in Protest: Environmental illness and the struggle over medical knowledge*, New York: New York University Press.

Kulenkampff, M., Schwartzman, J.S., Wilson, J. (1974) 'Neurological complications of pertussis inoculation', *Archives of Disease in Childhood*; 49: 46–9.

Kurlan, R. (1998) 'Tourette's syndrome and "Pandas": Will the relation bear out?', *Neurology*; 50 (6) (June): 1530–4.

*Lancet* (2000) 'Measles, MMR and autism: the confusion continues', (Editorial), *Lancet*; 355: 1379.

Leask, J.-A., Chapman, S. (1998) 'An attempt to swindle nature', press anti-immunisation reportage, 1993–97, *Australia and New Zealand Journal of Public Health*; 22: 17–26.

Leask, J.-A., Chapman, S., Hawe, P. (2000) 'The facts are not enough', *British Medical Journal*; (Rapid Responses) 25 January (www.bmj.com).

LeCouteur, A. (2003) *National Autism Plan for Children: Plan for the identification, assessment, diagnosis and access to early interventions for pre-school and primary school-aged children with autism spectrum disorders*, National Initiative for Autism: Screening and Assessment, London: National Autistic Society.

LeCouteur, A. et al (1988) 'Infantile autism and urinary excretion of peptides and protein-associated peptide complexes', *Journal of Autism and Developmental Disorders*; 18 (2) (June): 181–90.

Leese, B., Bosanquet, N. (1992) 'Immunization in the UK: policy review and future economic options', *Vaccine*; 10 (8): 491–9.

Legal Services Commission (2003) 'Decision to remove funding for MMR litigation upheld on appeal', press release, 11 September, see also 'Decision to remove funding for MMR litigation', transcript, 6 October 2003 at www.mmrthefacts.nhs.uk/news

Levitt, N. (1999) *Prometheus Bedevilled: Science and the contradictions of contemporary culture*, New Jersey: Rutgers.

Licinio, J., Alvarado, I., Wong, M-L. (2002) 'Autoimmunity in autism', (Editorial), *Molecular Psychiatry*, 7: 329.

Lindley, K.J., Milla, P.J., (1998) 'Autism, inflammatory bowel disease, and MMR vaccine' (Correspondence), *Lancet*, 351: 907.

McCormick, M.C. (2001) 'Public briefing/Opening Statement', 23 April, Committee on Immunization Safety Review, at www4.nationalacademies.org/news/nsf.

McNeil, D.G. (2002) 'When parents say no to child vaccinations', *New York Times*, 30 November.

McNeil, W.H. (1976) *Plagues and Peoples*, Harmondsworth: Penguin.

McTaggart, L. (1996) *What Doctors Don't Tell You: The truth about the dangers of modern medicine*, London: Harper Collins.

McTaggart, L. (ed) (2000) *The Vaccination Bible: The real risks they don't tell you about all the major vaccines*, London: Harper Collins.

Madsen, K.M., Hvidd, A., Vestergaard, M., Schendel, D., Wohlfart, J., Thorsen, P., Olsen, J., Melbye, M. (2002) 'A population-based study of MMR vaccine and autism', *New England Journal of Medicine*; 347: 1477–82.

Makela, A., Nuorti, J.P., Peltola, H. (2002) 'Neurologic disorders after MMR vaccination', *Pediatrics*, 110 (5): 957–63.

Malik, K. (1996) *The Meaning of Race: Race, history and culture in Western society*, London: Macmillan.

Mander, R. (2004) *Men and Maternity*, London: Routledge.

Marsh, B. (2003) 'Evidence of MMR risk is "compelling"', *Daily Mail*, 4 October.

Martin, E. (1994) *Flexible Bodies: The role of immunity in American culture from the days of polio to the age of Aids*, Boston, MA: Beacon Press.

Marx, K. (1894) *Capital: A critique of political economy*, Volume 3, (1959 edn) London: Lawrence and Wishart.

MCA/CSM (Medicines Control Agency/Committee on Safety of Medicines) (1999a) 'Report of the Working Party on MMR', at www.mca.gov.uk.

MCA/CSM (1999b) 'The safety of MMR vaccine', *Current Problems in Pharmacovigilance*; 25: 9–10.

MCA/DH (2001) 'Combined MMR vaccines: response of the MCA and the DoH to issues raised in papers published in *Adverse Drug Reactions and Toxicological Reviews*, 2000, 19.

Medicines and Healthcare Products Regulatory Agency (MHRA) (2003) 'Statement on safety of MMR vaccine by Geier and Geier – conclusions are not justified', London: MHRA.

Meszaros, J.R., Asch, D.A., Baron, J., Hershey, J.C., Kunreuther, H., Schwartz-Buzaglo, J. (1996) 'Cognitive processes and the decisions of some parents to forego pertussis vaccination for their children', *Journal of Clinical Epidemiology*; 49: 697–703.

Metcalf, J. (1998) 'Is measles infection associated with Crohn's disease? The current evidence does not support a causal link', *British Medical Journal*; 316: 166.

Miller, D.L., Madge, N., Diamond, J., Wadsworth, J., Ross, E. (1993) 'Pertussis immunisation and serious acute neurological illnesses in children', *British Medical Journal*, 307: 1171–6.

Miller, D.L., Ross, E.M., Alderslade, R., Bellman, M.H., Rawson, N.S.B. (1981) 'Pertussis immunisation and serious acute neurological illness in children', *British Medical Journal*; 282: 1595–9.

Miller, E., Andrews, N. (2001) 'Comments on "MMR: through a glass darkly"' (www.phls.co.uk/facts/Vaccination/012201wakefield.htm).

Miller, E., Farrington, P. (2000) 'Written testimony to the Congress of the United States House of Representatives Committee on Government Reform: Hearing on "The challenges of autism. Why the increased rates?"', April, at web.archive.org/web/200111116055137/www.house.gov/reform/hearings/healthcare/00.

Miller, E., Goldacre, M., Pugh, S. (1993) 'Risk of aseptic meningitis after MMR vaccine in UK children', *Lancet*; 341: 979–82.

Miller, E., Andrews, N., Waight, P., Taylor, B. (2003) 'Bacterial infections, immune overload, and MMR vaccine', *Archives of Disease in Childhood*; 88: 222–3.

Miller, E., Waight, P., Farrington, C.P., Andrews, N., Stowe, J., Taylor, B. (2001) 'Idiopathic thrombocytopenic purpura and the MMR vaccine', *Archives of Disease in Childhood*; 84: 227–9.

Mills, H. (2002) *MMR: The story so far*, *Private Eye* Special Report, London: *Private Eye*.

Mitchell, L. (2000) 'Secrets and lies: is the astonishing rise in autism a medical mystery or a pharmaceutical shame?' *Salon.com*, at archive.salon.com/mwt/feature/2000/08/02/autism/print.html.

Moses, V. (2002) 'Chewing over GM food', *spiked-online*, 5 February, www.spiked-online.com/Articles/00000002D3EF.htm.

Moulin, A.-M. (1989) 'Immunology old and new: the beginning and the end', in P. Mazumdar (ed) *Immunology 1930–1980: Essays on the history of immunology*, Toronto: Wall & Thompson.

MRC (Medical Research Council) (1998) 'Group concluded no reason for change in MMR vaccine policy', Press Release Ref: 09/98, London: MRC.

MRC (2000) 'Report of the strategy development group subgroup on research into inflammatory bowel disease and autism', March, at www.mrc.ac.uk.

MRC (2001) *Review of Autism Research: Epidemiology and Causes*, December, London: MRC.

Muir Gray, J.A. (1999) 'Post-modern medicine', *Lancet*; 354: 1552.

Murch, S. (2003) 'Separating inflammation from speculation in autism', (Correspondence), *Lancet*; 362: 1498–9.

Murch, S., Thomson, M., Walker-Smith, J.A. (1998) 'Autism, inflammatory bowel disease, and MMR vaccine', (Correspondence: authors' reply), *Lancet*; 351: 908.

Murch, S., Anthony, A., Casson, D.H., Malik, M., Berelowitz, M., Dhillon, A.P., Thomson, M., Valentine, A., Davies, S.E., Walker-Smith, J.A. (2004) 'Retraction of an interpretation', *Lancet*; 363 (6 March): 750.

Murphy, M.L., Pichichero, M.E. (2002) 'Prospective identification and treatment of children with paediatric autoimmune neuropsychiatric disorder associated with group A streptococcal infection', *Archives of Pediatrics and Adolescent Medicine*; 156 (4) (April): 356–61.

NAS (National Autistic Society) (2002) 'MMR: the NAS position', press statement, 12 March at www.nas.org.uk/.

NAS (2003) *Approaches to Autism: An easy to use guide to many and varied approaches to autism*, revised and updated, London: NAS.

National Research Council (2001) *Educating Young Children with Autism*, Washington, DC: National Academy Press.

National Statistics (2003) *Social Trends*; 33, Stationery Office (www.statistics.gov.uk/)

New York State Department of Health (1999) *Report of the Recommendations: Clinical Practice Guidelines, Autism/Pervasive Development Disorders, Assessment and Intervention for Young Children (Age 0–3 Years)* at www.health.state.ny.us/nydoh/eip/autism.htm.

Nicholson, R. (1994a) 'Measles and deception', *Bulletin of Medical Ethics*, August: 3–9.

Nicholson, R. (1994b) 'Is your measles jab really necessary?', *Bulletin of Medical Ethics*, October: 3–5.

Nicoll, A., Elliman, D., Ross, E. (1998) 'MMR vaccination and autism 1998: *British Medical Journal*, 316: 715–16.

Nicolson, P. (2002) *Having it all? Choices for today's superwoman*, London: John Wiley.

Noble, K.K., Miyasaka, K. (2003) 'MMR vaccine and autism' (Letter), *New England Journal of Medicine*; 348 (10): 952–3.

NVIC (National Vaccination Information Centre) (2000) See www.909shot.com/Conferences/Conferences.htm.

Offit, P.A. (2000) 'Autism – present challenges, future needs: why the increased rates?', Testimony to the Government Reform Committee, 6 April, at www.house.gov/reform/hearings/healthcare.

Offit, P.A. (2002) 'Vaccines and autism', Immunisation Action Coalition, www.immunize.org/catg.d/p2065.pdf.

Offit, P.A., Quarles, J., Gerber, M.A., Hackett, C.J., Marcuse, E.K., Kollman, T.R., Gellin, B.G., Landry, S. (2002) 'Addressing parents' concerns: do multiple vaccines overwhelm or weaken the infant's immune system?', Pediatrics; 109; 124–9, www.pediatrics.org/cgi/content/full/109/ 1/124.

Olby, R.C. (1999) 'Constitutional and hereditary diseases', in W.F. Bynum, R. Porter (eds) Companion Encyclopedia of the History of Medicine, Volume I, London: Routledge.

O'Leary, J.J. (2002a) 'Link found between measles virus and gut abnormalities in children with developmental disorder' (Press Statement), (see mp.bmjjournals.com/cgi/content/full/54/DC1).

O'Leary, J.J. (2002b) 'Neither this publication nor any public presentation by me or my research team has stated that MMR causes autism' (Press Statement, 16 June), (see www.mmrthefacts.nhs.uk/news).

O'Neill, O. (2002) Autonomy and Trust in Bioethics, Cambridge: Cambridge University Press.

Orenstein, A.O., Hinman, A.R. (1999) 'The immunisation system in the United States – the role of school immunisation laws', Vaccine; 17: S9–S24.

Pangborn, J.B., Baker, S.M. (2001) Biomedical Assessment Options for Children with Autism and Related Problems: A consensus report of the Defeat Autism Now (DAN!) Scientific Effort, San Diego, CA: Autism Research Institute.

Panksepp, J. (1979) 'A neurochemical theory of autism', Trends in Neuroscience; 2: 174–7.

Patja, A., Davidkin, I., Kurki, T., Kallio, M.J.T., Valle, M.H.P. (2000) 'Serious adverse events after MMR vaccination during a 14-year prospective follow-up', Pediatric Infectious Disease Journal; 19: 1127–34.

Pavone, L., Fiumara, A., Bottaro, G., Mazzone, D., Coleman, M. (1996) 'Autism in coeliac disease: failure to validate the hypothesis that a link might exist', Biological Psychiatry; 72–5.

Peckham, C. et al (1989) National Immunisation Study: Factors influencing immunisation uptake in childhood (Peckham Report), London: Institute of Child Health/Action Research for the Crippled Child.

Peltola, H., Davidkin, I., Valle, M., Paunio, M., Hovi, T., Heinonen, O.P., Leinikki, P. (1997) 'No measles in Finland', Lancet; 350: 1364–5.

Peltola, H. et al (2000) 'Mumps and rubella eliminated from Finland', Journal of the American Medical Association; 284: 2643–7.

Peltola, H., Patja, A., Leinikki, P., Valle, M., Davidkin, I., Paunio, M. (1998) 'No evidence for MMR vaccine-associated inflammatory bowel disease or autism in a 14-year prospective study', Lancet; 351: 1327–8.

Perlmutter, S.J., Leitman, S.F., Garvey, M.A., Hamburger, S., Feldman, S., Leonard, H.L. (1999) 'Therapeutic plasma exchange and intravenous immunoglobulin for obsessive-compulsive disorder and tic disorders in childhood', Lancet; 354: 1153–8.

Phillips, M. (2000) *Report of the BSE Inquiry*, Phillips Report, at www.bse.inquiry.gov.uk/.

Phillips, M. (2003) 'MMR: the truth', *Daily Mail*, 11–13 March.

Phillips, M. (2004) 'Why I believe Dr Wakefield was shamefully smeared', *Daily Mail*, 23 February.

Picardie, J. (2002) 'Special Report', *Daily Telegraph* (magazine), 8 June.

Pollak, R. (1996) *The Creation of Dr B: A biography of Bruno Bettelheim*, New York: Simon & Schuster.

Porter, M. (2003) 'Measles and the MMR jab', *The Scotsman*, 21 October, www.news.scotsman.com/archive.cfm?id=1160682003.

Preston, N.W. (1980) 'Whooping cough immunisation: fact and fiction', *Public Health London*, 94: 350–5.

Ramsay, M., Gay, N., Miller, E., Rush, M., White, J., Morgan-Capner, P., Brown, D. (1994) 'The epidemiology of measles in England and Wales: rationale for the 1994 national vaccination campaign', *Communicable Disease Report*; 4: R141–6.

*Private Eye* (2004) 'MMR: interesting conflicts', *Private Eye*, 1101 (5–18 March): 27.

Reichelt, K.L., Hole, K., Hamberger, A. (1993) 'Biologically active peptide-containing fractions in schizophrenia and childhood autism', *Advances in Biochemical Psychopharmacology*; 28: 627–43.

Reichelt, K.L., Knivsberg, A.M., Lind, G., Nodland,M. (2001) 'The probable etiology and possible treatment of childhood autism', *Brain Dysfunction*; 4: 308–19.

Richmond, P., Goldblatt, D. (1998) 'Autism, inflammatory bowel disease, and MMR vaccine' (Correspondence), *Lancet*; 351: 1355.

Rimland, B. (1965) *Infantile Autism: The syndrome and its implications for a neural theory of behaviour*, London: Methuen.

Rimland, B. (1998a) 'Vaccinations: the overlooked factors' at www.autism.com/ari/editorials/vaccinations.html.

Rimland, B. (1998b) 'The autism–secretin connection', *Autism Research Review International*; 12 (3): 3.

Rimland, B. (1999) Interview with Eileen Hopkins, www.autismconnect.org/interviews/transcripts/bernard_rimland.htm.

Rimland, B. (2002) 'The DAN! philosophy', www.autism.com/ari/dan statement.html

Roberts, G. (1999) 'MMR vaccination and autism' (Correspondence), *Lancet*; 354: 951.

Roberts, Y. (1995) 'A shot in the dark', *Sunday Times Magazine*, 17 December.

Rodier, P.M. (2000) 'The early origins of autism', *Scientific American*; 282 (2): 56–63.

Rogers, A. (2000) 'MMR litigation – clinical comment', *Medical Litigation*, October.

Rogers, A., Pilgrim, D. (1994) 'Rational non-compliance with childhood immunisation: personal accounts of parents and primary health care professionals', in Health Education Authority (ed) *Uptake of Immunisation: issues for health education*, London: Health Education Authority.

Rogers, A., Pilgrim, D. (1995) 'The risk of resistance: perspectives on the mass childhood immunisation programme', in J. Gabe (ed) *Medicine, Health and Risk: Sociological approaches*, Oxford: Blackwell.

Roth, I. (2002) 'The autistic spectrum: from theory to practice', in N. Brace, H. Wescott (eds) *Applying Psychology*, Milton Keynes: Open University.

Sabra, A., Bellanti, J.A., Colon, A.R. (1998) 'Ileal-lymphoid-nodular hyperplasia, non-specific colitis, and pervasive developmental disorder in children', (Correspondence), *Lancet*, 352: 234–5.

Sackett, D.L, Haynes, R.B., Guyatt, G.H., Tugwell, P. (1991) *Clinical Epidemiology: A basic science for clinical medicine*, second edn, Boston, MA/London/Toronto: Little, Brown.

Sacks, O. (1973) *Awakenings*, London: Duckworth.

Sacks, O. (1995) *An Anthropologist on Mars*, London: Picador.

Salisbury, D.M., Horsley, S.D. (1995) 'Measles campaign', *British Medical Journal*; 310: 1334.

Sandler, A.D., Sutton, K.A., DeWeese, J., Girardi, M.A., Sheppard, M.A., Bodfish, J.W. (1999) 'Lack of benefit of a single dose of synthetic human secretin in the treatment of autism and pervasive developmental disorder', *New England Journal of Medicine*; 341: 1801–6.

Schopler, E. (1996) 'Collaboration between research professional and consumer', *Journal of Autism and Developmental Disorders*; 26 (2): 277–80.

Scottish Executive (2002) *Recommendations of the MMR expert group*, www.scotland.gov.uk/library5/health/rmmr-13.asp.

Seroussi, K. (2000) 'Listen to the parents', *Looking Up Autism: International Newsletter*; 2 (3).

Shah, R.R. (2001) 'Thalidomide, drug safety and early drug regulation in the UK', *Adverse Drug Reactions and Toxicology Reviews*; 20 (4): 199–255.

Sharp, L.K., Wolfe, R.M. (2002) 'Antivaccinationists past and present', *British Medical Journal*, 325: 430–2.

Shattock, P. (1995) 'Back to the future: an assessment of some of the unorthodox forms of biomedical intervention currently being applied to autism', paper presented at the Durham Conference 1995, osiris. sunderland.ac.uk/autism/durham95.html.

Shattock, P. (1999) 'The use of secretin for the treatment of autism', osiris.sunderland.ac.uk/autism/sec.htm.

Shattock, P., Savery, D. (1997) *Autism as a Metabolic Disorder*, Sunderland: Autism Research Unit.

Shaw, W. (2002) *Biological Treatments for Autism and PDD*, Kansas: Great Plains Laboratory.

Shiels, O., Smyth, P., Martin, C., O'Leary, J.J. (2002) 'Development of an "allelic discrimination" type assay to differentiate between the strain origins of measles virus detected in intestinal tissue of children with ileocolonic lymphonodular hyperplasia and concomitant developmental disorder'. Abstract (No 20) presented at Pathological Society of Great Britain and Ireland (www.pathsoc.org.uk/meet/prog.shtml).

Singer, H.S. (1999) 'Pandas and immunomodulatory therapy', *Lancet*; 354: 1137–8.

Singh, V.K. (1999) 'Autism, autoimmunity and immunotherapy: a commentary', *Autism Autoimmunity Project Newsletter*; 1 (2) (December).

Singh, V.K. (2000) 'Autoimmunity and neurological disorders' (Interview), *Latitudes*; 4 (2), Association for Comprehensive Neurotherapy (at www.latitudes.org).

Singh, V.K., Lin, S.X., Yang, V.C. (1998) 'Serological association of measles virus and human herpesvirus-6 with brain autoantibodies in autism', *Clinical Immunology and Immunopathology*; 89 (October): 105–8.

Singh, V.K., Lin, S.X., Nelson, C. (2002) 'Abnormal measles–mumps–rubella antibodies and CNS autoimmunity in children with autism', *Journal of Biomedical Science*; 9 (4) (July-August): 359–64.

Southwood, R. (1989) *Report of the Working Party on Bovine Spongiform Encephalopathy*, London: HMSO.

Spectrum Interview (2000) 'So what's not to like about Andrew Wakefield?', (interview at the Autism 2000 conference, Kamloops, BC, at www.autismspectrum.com/vaccine.htm).

Spitzer, W.O. (2001a) 'A sixty day war of words: is MMR linked to autism?', *Adverse Drug Reactions and Toxicology Reviews*; 20 (1): 47–55.

Spitzer, W.O., Aitken, K.J., Dell'Aniello, S., Davis, M.W.L. (2001b) 'The natural history of autistic syndrome in British children exposed to MMR' *Adverse Drug Reactions and Toxicology Reviews*; 20 (3): 47–55.

Stephens, T., Brynner, R. (2001) *The Impact of Thalidomide and its Revival as a Vital Medicine*, Cambridge, MA: Perseus.

Stuart-Smith, L.J. (1988) *Loveday v Renton and Another*, Queen's Bench Division, *The Times* 31 March 1988, No 1982 L 1812 (Transcript: Clinton Vint).

Sumner (2003) Judgment between A&D and B&E, neutral citation number [2003] WEHC 1376 (Fam) at www.bailii.org/ew/cases/EWHC/Fam/2003/1376.html.

*Sunday Times* Insight Team (1979) *Suffer the Children: The story of thalidomide*, London: Futura.

Swales, J.D. (1992) 'The Leicester anti-vaccination movement', *Lancet*; 340: 1019–21.

Taylor, B. (2000) 'Testimony to the Congress of the United States House of Representatives Committee on Government Reform: Hearing on "The challenges of autism. Why the increased rates?"', 6 April, at web.archive.org/web/200111116055137/www.house.gov/reform/hearings/healthcare/00.

Taylor, B., Miller, E., Farrington, C.P. (1999b) 'MMR vaccination and autism', (Correspondence: authors' reply), *Lancet*; 354: 950.

Taylor, B., Miller, E., Lingam, R., Andrews, N., Simmons, A., Stowe, J. (2002) 'MMR vaccination and bowel problems or developmental regression in children with autism: population study', *British Medical Journal*; 324: 393–6.

Taylor, B., Miller, E., Farrington, C.P., Petropoulos, M.-C., Favot-Mayaud, I., Li, J., Waight, P.A. (1999a) 'Autism and MMR vaccine: no epidemiological evidence for a causal association', *Lancet*; 353: 2026–9.

Templeton, S.K. (2002) 'Triple jag autism could be next BSE' at www.whale.to/v//mmrbse.htm.

Thomson, N.P., Montgomery, S.M., Pounder, R.E., Wakefield, A.J. (1995) 'Is measles vaccination a risk factor for IBD?', *Lancet*, 345: 1071–4.

Thorpe, Sedley, Evans (2003) B (Child), Neutral Citation Number: [2003] EWCA Civ 1148 at www.bailii.org/ew/cases/EWCA/Civ/2003/1148.html.

Tilton, A.J. (2000) 'Transfer factor: immunotherapy for autism', *What you need to know about autism/pervasive developmental disorders*, autism.about.com/library/weekly/aa092700a.htm.

Tinbergen, N., Tinbergen, E. (eds) (1983), *Autistic Children: New hope for a cure*, London: Allen & Unwin.

Tommey, J. (2002a) 'Summary of biological problems', *Autism File*; 10.

Tommey, J. (2002b) 'Acquired autism', *Autism File*; 1–5 (compilation issue).

Tommey, J., Tommey, P. (2002) 'Foreword'; 1–5 (compilation issue).

Tommey, P. (2002) 'Comment', *Autism File*; 10.

Torrente, F. et al (2002) 'Small intestinal enteropathy with epithelial IgG and complement deposition in children with regressive autism', *Molecular Psychiatry*, 7 (4): 375–82.

Toynbee, P., Walker, D. (2001) *Did things get better? An audit of Labour's successes and failures*, London: Penguin.

Trevarthen, C., Aitken, K., Papoudi, D., Robarts, J. (1996) *Children with Autism: Diagnosis and intervention to meet their needs*, London: Jessica Kingsley.

Uhlmann, V., Shiels, O., Wakefield, A.J., O'Leary, J. (2002) 'Potential viral pathogenic mechanism for new variant IBD', *Journal of Clinical Pathology and Molecular Pathology*; 55 (2): 84–90.

Volkmar, F.R. (1999) 'Lessons from secretin', (Editorial), *New England Journal of Medicine*: 341: 1842–5.

Wakefield, A. (2004) 'A statement by Andrew Wakefield', *Lancet*; 363 (6 March): 823–4.

Wakefield, A.J. (1998) 'Autism, inflammatory bowel disease, and MMR vaccine', (Correspondence: author's reply), *Lancet*, 351: 908.

Wakefield A.J. (2001a) 'Killing the messenger: Dr Andrew Wakefield fired' (autism.about/com/library/weekly/aa120501a.htm).

Wakefield, A.J. (2001b) 'Testimony of Dr Andrew J Wakefield before the Government Reform Committee of the US House of Representatives', at www.unlockingautism.org/testimonies/index.

Wakefield, A.J. (2002a) 'Testimony of Dr Andrew J Wakefield', Committee on Government Reform (US House of Representatives), June 2002, (www.house.gov/reform/hearings/healthcare/02.06.19/wakefield.htm).

Wakefield, A.J. (2002b) *Visceral*, Press release, November, in response to Madsen et al (2002) at www.visceral.org.uk.

Wakefield, A.J. (2002c) 'Open letter to the editor of the *New England Journal of Medicine*', November, at www.freewebz.com/schafer/wakefield.htm.

Wakefield, A.J. (2002d) 'Enterocolitis, autism and measles virus', *Molecular Psychiatry*; 7 Suppl 2: S44–6.

Wakefield, A.J. (2002e) 'The gut–brain axis in childhood developmental disorders', *Journal of Pediatric Gastroenterology and Nutrition*; 34: S14–S17.

Wakefield, A.J., Montgomery, S.M. (1999) 'Autism, viral infection and the gut-brain axis', paper submitted to Autism99 internet conference at trainland.tripod.com/andrewj.htm.

Wakefield A.J., Montgomery, S.M. (2000) 'MMR vaccine: through a glass darkly', *Adverse Drug Reactions and Toxicology Reviews*; 19: 265–83.

Wakefield, A.J., Pittilo, R.M., Sim, R. (1993) 'Evidence of persistent measles virus infection in Crohn's disease', *Journal of Medical Virology*; 39: 345–53.

Wakefield, A.J., Puleston, J.M., Montgomery, S.M., Anthony, A., O'Leary, J.J., Murch, S.M. (2002) 'Review article: the concept of entero-colonic encephalopathy, autism and opioid receptor ligands', *Aliment Pharmacology Therapy*; 16: 663–74.

Wakefield A.J., Anthony, A., Murch, S.M., Thomson, M., Montgomery, S.M., Davies, S., O'Leary, J.J., Berelowitz, M., Walker-Smith, J.A. (2000) 'Enterocolitis in children with developmental disorders', *American Journal of Gastroenterology*; 95 (9): 2285–95.

Wakefield A.J., Murch, S.M., Anthony, A., Linnell, D.M., Casson, D.M., Malik, M., Berelowitz, M., Dhillon, A.P., Thomson, M.A., Harvey, P., Valentine, A., Davies, S.E., Walker-Smith, J.A. (1998) 'Ileal-lymphoid-nodular hyperplasia, non-specific colitis, and pervasive developmental disorder in children', *Lancet*; 351: 637–41.

Wakefield, A.J., Dhillon, A.P., Rowles, P.M., Sawyerr, A.M., Pittilo, R.M., Lewis, A.A.M., Pounder, R.E. (1989) 'Pathogenesis of Crohn's disease: multifocal gastrointestinal infarction', *Lancet* (4 November): 1057–62.

Wainwright, D., Calnan, M. (2002) *Work Stress: The making of a modern epidemic*, Buckingham/Philadelphia: Open University Press.

Walker, D.R. (1998) 'Autism, inflammatory bowel disease, and MMR vaccine' (Correspondence), *Lancet*; 351: 1355.

Walker-Smith, J.A. (1998) 'Autism, inflammatory bowel disease, and MMR vaccine' (Correspondence), *Lancet*; 351: 1356–7.

Walker-Smith, J.A. (2003) *Enduring Memories: A paediatric gastroenterologist remembers*, London: The Memoir Club.

Wessely, S., Hotopf, M., Sharpe, M. (1998) *Chronic Fatigue and its Syndromes*, Oxford: Oxford University Press.

Whiteley, P., Shattock, P. (1997) *Guidelines for the Implementation of a Gluten and/or Casein-free Diet with People with Autism or Associated Spectrum Disorders*, Sunderland: Autism Research Unit.

Wilson, K., Mills, E., Ross, C., McGowan, J., Jadad, A. (2003) 'Association of autistic spectrum disorder and MMR vaccine: a systematic review of current epidemiological evidence', *Archives of Pediatric and Adolescent Medicine*; 157: 628–34.

Wing, J.K. (ed) (1966) *Early Childhood Autism: Clinical, educational and social aspects*, Oxford: Pergamon.

Wing, L. (1966) 'Counselling parents', in Wing, J.K. (ed) *Early Childhood Autism: Clinical, educational and social aspects*, Oxford: Pergamon.

Wing, L. (ed) (1988) *Aspects of Autism: Biological Research*, London: Royal College of Psychiatrists.

Wing, L. (1996a) *The Autistic Spectrum: A guide for parents and professionals*, London: Constable.

Wing, L. (1996b) 'Autistic spectrum disorders: no evidence for an increase in prevalence', *British Medical Journal*, 312: 327–8.

Wing, L. (1997) 'The autistic spectrum', *Lancet*, 350: 1761–6.

Wing, L. (2001) 'My views on the existence of regressive autism', *Looking up Autism*; 2 (8).

Wing, L., Potter, D. (2002) 'The epidemiology of autistic spectrum disorders: is the prevalence rising?', *Mental Retardation and Developmental Disabilities Research Reviews*; 8 (3): 151–61.

Wolfe, R.M., Sharp, L.K. (2002) 'Anti-vaccinationists past and present', *British Medical Journal*; 325: 430–2.

Wolpert, L. (1992) *The Unnatural Nature of Science*, London: Faber.

Wonder, S (1972) *Superstition*, www.stevie-wonder.com

WHO (World Health Organization) (1998) 'Expanded programme on immunisation (EPI) – association between measles infection and the occurrence of chronic IBD', *Weekly Epidemiology Record*; 73: 33–40.

Zhang, J., Rivers, G., Peyser, J., Zack, B., Horvath, K., Rusche, J. (2000) 'Analysis of compounds in the urine of children with autism using HPLC-mass spectrometry', *Journal of Paediatric Gastroenterology and Nutrition*; 31 (Supp 12): 32.

# INDEX